The Healthy Heart Handbook

Flush Your Arteries, Heal Your Heart, and Lower High Blood Pressure, Without Dangerous Drugs or Risky Surgery

Publishers Note

This book is intended for general information only. It does not constitute medical, legal, or financial advice or practice. The editors of FC&A have taken careful measures to ensure the accuracy and usefulness of the information in this book. While every attempt has been made to ensure accuracy, errors may occur. Some websites, addresses, and telephone numbers may have changed since printing. We cannot guarantee the safety or effectiveness of any advice or treatments mentioned. Readers are urged to consult with their professional financial advisors, lawyers, and health care professionals before making any changes.

This book is intended for general information only. It does not constitute medical advise or practice. We cannot guarantee the safety or effectiveness of any treatment or advice mentioned. Readers are urged to consult with their health care professionals and get their approval before undertaking therapies suggested by information in this book, keeping in mind that errors in the text may occur as in all publications and that new findings may supercede older information.

Peace I leave with you; my peace I give you. I do not give to you as the world gives. Do not let your hearts be troubled and do not be afraid.

John 14:27

Contents

Heart smarts

Beginner's guide to better health .1

How your heart works 2

What you need to know about cholesterol 3

7 reliable ways to lower your blood pressure 7

9 common signs of a heart attack 9

Ease the squeeze of angina pain 12

Can coughing save your life? 14

Know the symptoms of a stroke 15

New theory about heart disease 18

Strategies to determine your heart disease risk 21

High-tech ways to ward off a heart attack 27

Angioplasty or coronary bypass surgery – which is better? . .30

Find the best hospital for heart surgery 33

Straight talk about dangerous hospital infections 34

Survival guide for leg cramp sufferers 37

Triumph over congestive heart failure 40

5 ways to fight congestive heart failure 43

Help your heart keep the beat .45

Cut your risk of 'sudden death' 47

Prescription drugs

The good and the bad 49

ACE heart health and strengthen blood vessels 50

Slash bad cholesterol with statins 53

2 easy ways to save on statin drugs 56

Know your alternatives 58

Get the real story on aspirin 60

Avoid a prescription for disaster 62

7 questions to ask your doctor about a new Rx 64

Get the facts about HRT and your heart 66

Nutrition know-how

Take a bite out of heart disease 69

'Super foods' that heal your heart 70

19 natural ways to lower your cholesterol 70

Focus on fats to beat artery-clogging cholesterol 72

Ancient oil keeps arteries clean 75

Tiny seeds fight the 'Big Three' 77

Great reasons to eat more nuts 80

Fishy solution for a healthy heart 85

Avocados – armor for your heart 86

Cut LDL with a butter knife 89

Nutritional superhero to the rescue 92

A sweet treat that heals your heart 95

Nutritional powerhouse great for snacking 98

4 great reasons to eat whole grains 101

A better way to cut cholesterol 103

Healthy breakfast fights heart disease 106

Sweep out cholesterol with wheat germ 107

An apple a day keeps heart disease at bay 110

Pick the best proteins 111

'Cheap' way to clobber cholesterol 114

Enjoy the health benefits of the Asian diet 116

Antioxidants – secret weapons stop cell damage 118

Tart berry guards your arteries 119

Powerful brew renews blood vessels 121

Juicy fruit fends off illness 123

Little fruit packs big punch .126

4 ways garlic keeps you healthy 129

Delicious drink fends off heart disease 131

Southern grapes good for the heart 132

Happy 'half-hour' might help your heart 133

A sweet way to boost good cholesterol 135

Behold the amazing benefits of blueberries 137

Tiny fruit puts the squeeze on plaque 141

Take a bite out of plaque buildup 142

Yummy spice cuts cholesterol and blood sugar 144

Shake your taste for salt 147

Spot hidden sources of salt .148

Sodium content of common foods 150

Eat less sodium to keep more calcium 152

Salt substitute could save your life 153

DASH high blood pressure in 6 simple steps 154

Think like Popeye to K.O. high blood pressure 158

Pour yourself a cup of heart health 161

Reverse heart disease by this time next year 163

Forbidden food actually blocks cholesterol 166

2 steps toward lower cholesterol 168

Diet defense

8 weeks to a healthier mind and body 171

Feel younger, healthier, and more energetic 172

Turn back the clock with water 173

Drink up and reap the rewards 173

How much water should you drink? 174

Contents

Not all waters are created equal 176

Guard against health problems with grains 176

Maximize benefits with whole grains 177

Why you need more fiber 178

Dangerous dosage turns good vitamin bad 179

Balance blood sugar with chromium 181

Vital mineral for heart health 181

Age gracefully with fruits and veggies 182

Put the brakes on free radicals .183

Arm yourself with vitamin C 184

Defend your heart with phytochemicals 185

Color your world healthy with vitamin A 187

Keep your body moving with potassium 187

Keep breaks at bay with vitamin K 188

Stay stronger, longer with dairy 189

Count on calcium's many benefits 190

Strengthen your body with phosphorus 192

Defend your heart with vitamin D 192

Steer clear of saturated fat 193

7 easy ways to eat more dairy foods 194

Zap high cholesterol with legumes 194

Pack a powerful punch with protein 196

Muscle up with magnesium 197

Maximize energy with biotin 197

'Go fish' for heart health 198

Perk up your heart with polyunsaturated fats 199

Iron out weakness and fatigue .200

Strengthen your immune system with B6 201

Reel in better health with vitamin B12 202

Make zinc your link to wellness 203

Get the lowdown on nuts, seeds, and meats 204

Squirrel away nutritious nuts and seeds 205

Heal your heart with monounsaturated fat 206

Give bad cholesterol the boot with vitamin E 206

The truth about meat 208

Sweets and snacks survival guide 209

Think 'natural' to satisfy a sweet tooth 210

Get the skinny on fats 212

4 golden rules of good nutrition 213

Exercise your heart muscle

Simple steps to a stronger heart 215

Build a stronger heart for a longer life 216

Exercise makes you 'young-at-heart' 218

Endurance-level exercise benefits heart 221

Improve your endurance with exercise 223

Examples of endurance activities 226

Unbeatable way to reach your target 227

Sidestep deadly diseases 229

3 ways to get more gusto from your walk 230

Every step helps your heart 233

Fun way to flatten your belly 235

Reap big rewards in just 11 minutes twice a day 238

Guaranteed weight-loss secret 240

Best dieting tool – heart-healthy exercise 241

Lower blood pressure with gentle tai chi 243

Cycling your way to a better heart 244

Lighten up

Secrets to winning the battle of the bulge 247

Say goodbye to extra pounds for good 248

Lose weight without even trying 251

Wise up to dangers of popular diet plan 253

Make friends with healthy fats .256

7 secrets for a slimmer you 258

Diet pills you should know about 260

Straight talk about weight-loss scams 262

Super strategies for successful weight control 263

3 great reasons to eat more fiber 266

High-fiber recipes for healthy eating 267

7 ways fiber helps you win at losing 273

4 ways to shake off stress and lose weight 275

Dieting dozen gets the job done 277

Old world secret for a long life 280

Small changes help you take off pounds 284

Check out the only 'diet' you'll ever need 288

Get milk and get slim 290

Take a look at the latest food label lingo 293

Secret weapon in the war on fat 295

Get the skinny on popular diet plans 297

Back to basics – simple slimming solutions 298

12 smart ways to eat less fat 301

Think small for big changes 303

Dine out without throwing out your diet 304

Fool yourself into shedding pounds 307

5 clever ways to eat less 309

Dig up the 'dirt' on weight-loss gimmicks 311

Weigh the benefits of green tea 313

Powerful protectors

When diet and exercise aren't enough 315

Zap cholesterol with psyllium .316

6 secrets to buying safe and effective supplements 318

Net the benefits of fish oil supplements 321

Straight talk about a popular supplement 323

New hope for people with heart disease 325

Good ways – and bad ways – to boost your metabolism . .327

4 reasons to bypass red yeast rice 328

Boost heart health with pycnogenol 329

Ancient Asian remedy battles cholesterol 331

Keep the beat

Super solutions for a balanced life 333

Laugh your way to a healthy mind and body 334

26 proven, practical stress-busting tips 335

Fortify your health with optimism 339

Surprising stroke triggers 341

Ambush high blood pressure with close ties 342

Easy path to a healthy heart 344

Music keeps blood pressure in tune 345

Uncover a hidden threat to your heart 346

Fight depression to cut stroke risk 348

15 ways to stop smoking more easily 352

Guard your health with a pet 354

Put your worries to rest with prayer 355

6 ways to deal with anger 357

Secrets to keeping your heart safe in winter 358

Impotence: early warning sign of clogged arteries 360

Escape little-known heart danger 361

Index 363

Heart smarts

Beginner's guide to better health

How your heart works

Cal Ripken Jr. played in 2,632 consecutive baseball games. The late, great James Brown called himself the hardest-working man in show business. Yet, compared to your heart, they both look like slackers.

Your heart has an important job to do — pumping blood through your body — and this muscular organ never takes any time off. About the size of your fist, your heart weighs about 11 ounces and contains four chambers. The upper chambers, or atria, receive blood, while the lower chambers, or ventricles, pump blood out.

Veins carry oxygen-poor blood from the body to the right atrium. The blood then moves down into the right ventricle, which pumps the blood to the lungs, where it picks up oxygen. The oxygenated blood returns to the heart through the left atrium and moves down to the left ventricle, which pumps the oxygen-rich blood through the aorta. This main artery branches into smaller arteries and capillaries to deliver blood and oxygen to the rest of your body.

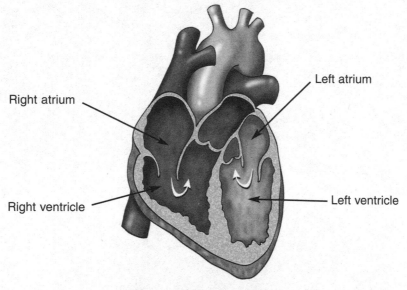

Right atrium

Left atrium

Right ventricle

Left ventricle

The heart's four chambers

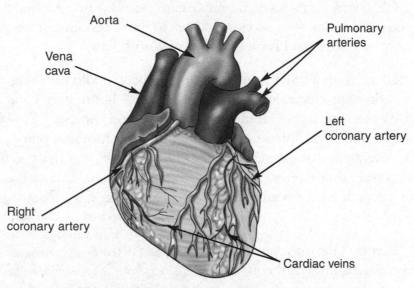

The heart's main arteries and veins

The cycle repeats itself as the oxygen-poor blood returns to your heart through your veins. Unfortunately, things do not always run smoothly.

Like your other organs, your heart needs the oxygen and nutrients that blood provides. That's why the coronary arteries, which deliver the oxygenated blood from the lungs to the heart, are so important. When these key arteries become clogged or blocked, you develop coronary artery disease, or heart disease.

High cholesterol, high blood pressure, and other conditions can take their toll on your heart and blood vessels. Unless you take the right steps, you could suffer a heart attack or stroke. Read on to discover what puts your heart at risk — and how to protect yourself.

What you need to know about cholesterol

Boo! Cholesterol has become something of a bogeyman, a scary, shadowy menace to fear. But cholesterol is much more complicated than that.

3

Cholesterol serves several important functions in your body. Your body needs this soft, waxy substance to make certain hormones, build cell walls, and form bile salts to absorb fats.

Foods from animal sources, including beef, poultry, fish, cheese, and dairy products, all contain cholesterol – but dietary cholesterol does not have as big an impact on your blood cholesterol as you might think. Saturated fat, the kind found in meat and dairy products, as well as some vegetable oils like palm oil and hydrogenated vegetable shortenings, has the biggest effect on your cholesterol levels.

> **atherosclerosis** collections of fatty deposits and fibrous tissue, known as plaques, that build up within the artery walls, narrowing your arteries and reducing the amount of blood that flows through them.

Diet isn't the only source of cholesterol, or even the main source for most people. Your liver manufactures cholesterol from other fats. There is a constant interchange of cholesterol between your liver and the rest of your body. To travel through your body, cholesterol needs some sort of transportation, so it hitches a ride with substances called lipoproteins. When people talk about the different types of cholesterol, they're actually talking about the different lipoproteins that carry it. Here's a quick look at the two main types.

▸ Low-density lipoprotein (LDL). Commonly called "bad" cholesterol, LDL transports cholesterol to your artery walls, where it can do damage.

▸ High-density lipoprotein (HDL). Known as "good" cholesterol, HDL whisks cholesterol from your bloodstream to your liver, where it becomes eliminated from your body.

Lowering your LDL cholesterol and boosting your HDL cholesterol can help reduce your risk of heart-related problems. LDL cholesterol plays a key role in the development of atherosclerosis and heart disease. In the past, cholesterol was thought to simply clog your arteries, like gunk clogging a pipe. While the process is more complicated than that, too much cholesterol still leads to dangerous blockages and blood clots.

You also need to worry about other lipids, or fats, in your blood called triglycerides. Like cholesterol, these fats show up in the foods you eat and serve a purpose in your body – but high levels mean trouble.

Unfortunately, you can't tell if you have high cholesterol or elevated triglycerides without getting a blood test. There are no outward symptoms until it's too late.

A standard lipid profile measures your total cholesterol and your levels of LDL, HDL, and triglycerides. You can get this simple blood test done at your doctor's office or local laboratory. Plan to get at least one lipid profile every five years.

Your total cholesterol should be below 200 milligrams per deciliter (mg/dL). Men should aim for HDL levels of 40 mg/dL or higher, while women should boost their HDL to 50 mg/dL or higher. Ideally, both men and women should have HDL levels of 60 mg/dL or higher.

In recent years, the guidelines for LDL cholesterol levels have changed. Your target LDL levels vary depending on your number of heart attack risk factors. The higher your risk, the lower your LDL needs to be.

- ▶ for those at low risk, below 160 mg/dL

- ▶ for people with two or more risk factors, less than 130 mg/dL with an optimal goal of less than 100 mg/dL

- ▶ for those with heart disease, other cardiovascular problems, or diabetes, less than 100 mg/dL with an optimal goal of 70 mg/dL

Risk factors include cigarette smoking, high blood pressure, low HDL cholesterol, and a family history of premature heart attacks. That means your father or brother had a heart attack before age 55 or your mother or sister had a heart attack before age 65. Men age 45 and older and women age 55 and older are also at greater risk.

Tame your triglycerides

Having high triglyceride levels increases your risk of heart disease. You can get your triglyceride levels measured during a normal cholesterol screening, or lipid profile. Here's what the numbers mean.

500 and above — very high

200–499 — high

150–199 — borderline high

below 150 — normal

Simple lifestyle changes, including a low-fat diet, weight loss, and exercise, can help lower triglycerides. You may also need to take medication.

Now that you know what numbers to strive for, how do you go about lowering your cholesterol?

The right diet is a good first step. Pay particular attention to the fats you eat. Saturated fats are the main culprit in raising cholesterol, but trans fats also do damage. These dangerous fats, found in processed foods and baked goods, may boost triglycerides and lower protective HDL cholesterol.

Choose healthier unsaturated fats instead. Monounsaturated fat, the kind found in olive oil, canola oil, avocados, and peanuts, and polyunsaturated fats, found in vegetable oils and fish, both make good choices.

Fat should make up no more than 20 to 35 percent of your daily calories, with no more than 7 percent coming from saturated fat. Protein should account for 15 percent, and carbohydrates should make up the remaining 55 percent.

Losing weight, quitting smoking, and becoming more active will also help. Even if you eat right, shed some pounds, and exercise regularly, you may still need cholesterol-lowering drugs, like statins, to help get your cholesterol down to a healthy level. For more information about statins, see "Slash bad cholesterol with statins" on page 53.

7 reliable ways to lower your blood pressure

Your heart works hard enough. Why make its job any harder? That's what happens when you have high blood pressure.

High blood pressure, or hypertension, not only makes your heart work harder to pump blood through your body, it also boosts your risk of heart attack, stroke, kidney disease, and blindness.

Measured in milligrams of mercury (mmHg), your blood pressure tells you the force of your blood against the walls of your arteries. Systolic blood pressure, the top number in a blood pressure reading, refers to the pressure when your heart contracts. Diastolic blood pressure, the bottom number, measures blood pressure when the heart relaxes between contractions.

Like high cholesterol, high blood pressure has no outward symptoms. That makes it essential to get your blood pressure checked by a doctor. Otherwise, you may not know you have high blood pressure until it's too late. Here's how to make sense of your blood pressure reading.

▶ Lower than 120/80 – normal.

▶ 120–139/80–89 – prehypertension. Think of a blood pressure reading in this range as a warning sign. You are at risk for developing high blood pressure unless you start taking steps to get it under control.

▶ 140/90 or higher – high blood pressure.

Blood pressure increases with age. In fact, two-thirds of Americans over age 60 have high blood pressure. Blacks may have greater risk than others. Being overweight and inactive, smoking, drinking, stress, and a diet high in salt and fat can also contribute to high blood pressure.

Your doctor may prescribe one or more medications to lower your blood pressure. But in many cases, you can get your blood pressure under control with a few simple lifestyle changes.

▶ Lose weight if you're overweight.

▶ Eat a healthy diet. Aim for more fruits, vegetables, and whole grains while cutting back on fat, red meat, and sweets – including sweetened drinks.

▶ Cut back on salt.

▶ Exercise regularly.

▶ Reduce stress.

▶ Quit smoking.

▶ Drink alcohol in moderation, if at all. This means no more than two drinks a day for a man and one for a woman.

Sticking to these simple lifestyle and dietary changes can dramatically lower your blood pressure – and help you avoid blood pressure medication entirely. That's what researchers discovered in the PREMIER study.

People in the study lost weight, exercised, reduced salt and alcohol intake, and followed the National Heart, Lung, and Blood Institute's Dietary Approaches to Stop Hypertension (DASH) diet – which emphasizes many of the dietary tips listed previously.

In the study, 98 percent of those with high blood pressure became completely free of their medicine when they followed this simple advice.

Simple tip for an accurate reading

Your doctor checks your blood pressure — but he can also affect it. Up to 35 percent of people with high blood pressure have a condition called "white coat hypertension." This means that your blood pressure is high when checked by a doctor or in a medical setting, but normal otherwise. Fortunately, you can buy a home monitor and check your blood pressure yourself. This will give you a more accurate measurement of your usual blood pressure. Having your blood pressure checked by a nurse rather than a doctor may also help.

9 common signs of a heart attack

A heart attack may strike suddenly, but it's an event years in the making. Atherosclerosis, or the buildup of plaque within the walls of your coronary arteries, is usually to blame. Plaque typically accumulates and pushes the inner wall of the artery inward, causing a "stenosis" or narrowing of the space where blood flows to supply the heart muscle. This constriction can cause heart pain or "angina."

The constriction may become severe enough by itself to cause a heart attack that sends the heart muscle into spasms that don't pump blood effectively. Also, the

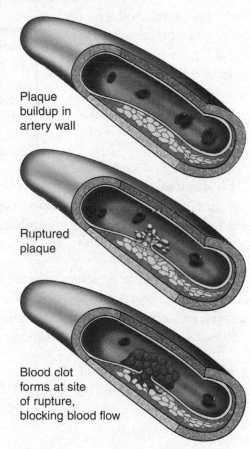

Plaque buildup in artery wall

Ruptured plaque

Blood clot forms at site of rupture, blocking blood flow

plaque inside the artery wall may rupture and spill its contents into the channel where blood flows, causing a blood clot to form that completely shuts off the flow of blood to the part of the heart muscle served by that artery.

This cuts off the blood supply to the myocardium, the muscular layer of the heart wall that helps the heart pump. Without the oxygen it needs, the heart muscle will die.

Quick emergency transportation to a hospital emergency room can be a lifesaver for heart attack victims. Every minute of delay increases risk of fatality.

A heart attack – also known as a myocardial infarction – can strike anyone, but older people and blacks are at greater risk. Other risk factors include a sedentary lifestyle, obesity, smoking, high blood pressure, high cholesterol, and a family history of heart attacks. Before age 50, men are more likely to have a heart attack than women – but, after menopause, women's risk increases as their levels of estrogen decrease.

> **heart attack** a sudden blockage of blood flow to the heart, usually due to a blood clot. Doctors may call it myocardial infarction. This blockage can kill heart tissue and damage your heart.

Heart attacks announce themselves in several ways. Do you know the nine signs of a heart attack in progress, or about to begin? This wisdom is essential for every family member of anyone who has high blood pressure.

The most common sign of a heart attack is crushing pain in your chest, which can radiate to your arms (especially your left arm), shoulders, neck, jaw, back, or abdomen. You may also feel a sense of fullness, squeezing, or pressure in your chest.

However, nearly half of all women and a third of all men feel no chest pain or discomfort at all during a heart attack. Often, women suffer from unusual fatigue, sleep disturbances, and shortness of breath for about a month before the heart attack.

Other signs of a heart attack include profuse sweating, lightheadedness, nausea, a feeling of heartburn, dizziness, and fainting.

Sudden heart attack? Not likely! Most struck by heart attacks have symptoms for up to an hour before. Know these life-saving signs to look for — and what to do.

If you experience any of these symptoms, call 911 right away. You may also want to chew an aspirin. Fast action can save your life and limit the damage to your heart.

Of course, the best strategy is to prevent a heart attack in the first place. Keep your heart in tip-top shape with these simple tips.

▶ Eat a healthy diet low in saturated fats and rich in fruits, vegetables, and whole grains.

▶ Exercise regularly. Aim for 30 minutes of moderate exercise a day.

▶ Lose weight if you're overweight.

▶ Keep your blood pressure and cholesterol levels within a healthy range.

▶ Quit smoking.

▶ Drink in moderation if you drink alcohol. That means two drinks a day for a man and one drink for a woman.

You may also want to ask your doctor about low-dose aspirin therapy. Taking an aspirin a day can help prevent heart attacks in men and in women over age 65. However, aspirin therapy is not for everyone. Aspirin increases the risk of intestinal bleeding and hemorrhagic stroke — dangers that may outweigh its benefits if you're not at high risk for a heart attack.

Be alert to heart attack symptoms to save a life

Many people — even those who have heart disease — don't know the signs of a heart attack. Call for emergency help if you or someone else experiences any of these symptoms:

▸ crushing pain in your chest, which can radiate to your arms, shoulders, neck, jaw, back, or abdomen

▸ fullness, squeezing, or pressure in your chest

▸ unusual fatigue or sleep disturbances

▸ shortness of breath

▸ profuse sweating

▸ lightheadedness

▸ nausea or heartburn

▸ dizziness

▸ fainting

Ease the squeeze of angina pain

Pain is never pleasant, but pain in your chest can be very scary. However, it doesn't always mean you're having a heart attack. Sometimes recurring chest pain is due to angina.

Angina is a symptom of too little blood getting to your heart. One of the most common culprits is coronary artery disease (CAD), when plaque builds up in your coronary arteries, which supply blood directly to your heart muscle.

The arteries become clogged, narrow, and stiff. Less blood reaches your heart muscle, so it doesn't get all the oxygen it needs. Uncontrolled high blood pressure and other types of heart disease can also lead to angina.

An angina attack can feel like a heart attack and be just as frightening. You may feel a pressing or squeezing type of pain, usually just under your breastbone. The pain may spread to your shoulders, neck, jaws, arms, or back.

Fortunately, unlike a heart attack, angina usually causes no permanent damage because blood flow is only partially cut off. In a heart attack, the blood supply to part of your heart is blocked completely, damaging your heart muscle beyond repair.

Stable angina, the most common kind, follows a pattern. It most often strikes after exercising, when your heart can't get enough oxygen. Emotional stress can set it off, too.

Heavy meals, alcohol, cigarette smoke, and extreme heat or cold might also trigger an attack. Generally, the pain goes away in a few minutes if you rest or take your angina medicine. While it's not an emergency, stable angina does raise your risk of a heart attack.

Unstable angina is more serious. It's caused by a blood clot partially or totally blocking an artery. If the clot is big enough, it will cause a heart attack. This type of angina does not follow a pattern or improve with rest or medication. Get medical help right away if you experience:

▶ angina pain while resting, or pain that wakes you up.

▶ sudden, moderate to severe angina pain when you have never had it before.

▶ a significant increase in frequency or severity of angina if you have had stable angina.

If you have angina, consider yourself fortunate in one respect. This condition may serve as a warning to take better care of your heart and your health to prevent more serious heart problems.

Drink alcohol only in moderation. One large study, the Physicians' Health Study of more than 22,000 male doctors, found that moderate drinking may protect against angina and heart attack.

13

Men who drank one alcoholic drink a day were less likely to experience angina or have a heart attack, compared to men averaging less than one. However, moderation is key. The same study also found an increased risk of cancer among men who consumed two or more alcoholic drinks a day. The adverse consequences of heavy drinking far outweigh any health benefit.

Eat small and light. You may not think digesting your food is a difficult chore, but heavy meals make your heart work harder and can make you more likely to have an angina attack. Try eating smaller, lighter meals and relaxing afterward.

Trim the fat. Excess weight can aggravate your angina. The more weight you carry around, the harder your heart has to work. Certain fats can also clog up your arteries, so try to stick to foods low in saturated and trans fats.

Get a little exercise. Ask your doctor what kinds of activity you can safely do. Slow down and take frequent breaks if exercise tends to trigger your angina.

Stop smoking. This bad habit further narrows your arteries, which only makes angina worse.

Learn to relax. Try to avoid stressful or upsetting situations if stress usually sets off an attack. Read up on relaxation techniques and ask your doctor about stress-management strategies.

Can coughing save your life?

During cardiac arrest, a few coughs just might be the difference between life and death. Coughing helps pump blood through the body and to the brain so you don't lose consciousness before help arrives.

At the first sign of trouble, cough forcefully every one to two seconds in sets of five coughs. The American Heart Association (AHA) does not endorse "cough CPR" or teach it as a technique in its CPR courses — not because it doesn't work, but because it only helps in rare instances. It's much more important to call 911 for emergency help at the first sign of a heart attack.

When to call 9-1-1

You've had angina attacks before, but this one is almost unbearable. Should you just grimace and endure the pain or head for the hospital? Here are some signs that you should seek emergency medical attention.

▶ extreme pain or discomfort that gets worse and lasts longer than 20 minutes

▶ pain or discomfort along with weakness, feeling sick to your stomach, or fainting

▶ pain or discomfort that does not go away when you take three nitroglycerin tablets

▶ pain or discomfort that is worse than you have ever had before

If you are experiencing any of these symptoms, call an ambulance or have someone drive you to the hospital. Do not attempt to drive yourself.

Know the symptoms of a stroke

Stroke, also called brain attack, ranks third behind only heart disease and cancer as a cause of death in the United States. Ischemic stroke, the most common type, occurs when a blood clot blocks blood vessels to the brain, cutting off the brain's supply of oxygen. In a hemorrhagic stroke, a blood vessel bursts, leading to bleeding in or around the brain.

Both types of strokes can have devastating results. Besides killing you, stroke can also affect your motor skills, speech, memory, behavior, senses, and thought processes depending on which parts of your brain are damaged.

Older people, blacks, men, and those with a family history of stroke are at higher risk. Other risk factors include high blood pressure, high cholesterol, heart disease, diabetes, smoking, and obesity.

When it comes to a stroke, every second counts. The longer oxygen remains cut off from your brain, the more damage occurs. Often, acting quickly can be the difference between life and death.

That's why it's so important to know the signs of a stroke and how to respond to a brain attack.

Symptoms of a stroke include sudden weakness or numbness of your face, arm, or leg, especially on one side of your body; confusion; trouble speaking or understanding; difficulty seeing; dizziness, loss of balance or coordination; and a sudden, severe headache.

Even if the symptoms pass quickly without any lasting effects, do not ignore them. It could be a transient ischemic attack, or TIA. These "mini-strokes" often come before a full-blown stroke, so they should be taken seriously. Think of them as a warning sign.

3 surefire signs of a stroke

When you suspect someone is having a stroke, ask the person these three simple questions:

▸ Can you smile?

▸ Can you raise both hands above your head?

▸ Can you speak a complete sentence?

If the person has trouble with any of these tasks, call 911.

If you think you – or someone else – may be having a stroke, call 911 right away. You can also drive the person to the hospital. But never let someone having a stroke drive himself – and never attempt to drive yourself if you are the one experiencing the stroke.

Once at the hospital, you'll get quick treatment. If you arrive within three hours of the start of an ischemic stroke, you may receive the emergency drug alteplase (Activase). Also called a tissue plasminogen activator (t-PA), this clot-busting drug can stop an ischemic stroke in progress. In the case of a hemorrhagic stroke, surgery may be necessary.

stroke the sudden loss of blood, oxygen, and nutrients to brain cells, leading to a loss of brain function. A "brain attack" occurs when an artery that supplies blood to your brain becomes blocked (ischemic stroke) or ruptures (hemorrhagic stroke).

Strokes are far from inevitable. In fact, more than half of all strokes could be prevented if people took the right measures. Here are some terrific tactics to sidestep stroke.

▸ Control high blood pressure. High blood pressure, the No. 1 risk factor for stroke, contributes to 70 percent of all strokes. Keep your blood pressure within a healthy range.

▸ Quit smoking. Smokers have a 50-percent greater risk of stroke than nonsmokers. Cigarettes boost your risk of both ischemic and hemorrhagic stroke. You should also do your best to avoid secondhand smoke.

▸ Lose weight. Obesity, especially abdominal obesity, dramatically boosts your risk of stroke. Cut back on calories and become more active to shed those extra pounds.

▸ Exercise regularly. Being a couch potato can triple your risk of stroke compared to people who are physically active. Exercise helps you overcome stroke risk factors, like obesity and high blood pressure. Aim for at least 30 minutes of activity a day.

▶ Avoid alcohol. Drinking moderately may reduce your risk of ischemic stroke, but it boosts your risk of hemorrhagic stroke. Heavy drinking causes several health problems that can increase your stroke risk.

▶ Improve your cholesterol. Boosting your HDL, or good, cholesterol can reduce your risk of stroke. So can lowering your total and LDL, or bad, cholesterol. Eat a healthy diet, exercise, and take cholesterol-lowering medication, if necessary, to achieve your goals.

Negative emotions, such as anger, fear, irritability, or nervousness, may also contribute to stroke. Find ways to stay calm or avoid stressful situations. Air pollution may also boost your risk of ischemic stroke, so moving from the city to the country may do some good.

Arm yourself with this lifesaver

You're having a stroke! But which kind? When you arrive at the hospital, your doctor should perform diagnostic tests, such as a CT scan, to determine whether your stroke is ischemic or hemorrhagic before administering clot-busting drugs or blood thinners. Skipping this step could lead to your death. If there's bleeding in your brain from a hemorrhagic stroke, these drugs will just make the bleeding worse. Armed with this lifesaving information, your doctor can take the appropriate steps to treat your stroke.

New theory about heart disease

Recently, a new theory has emerged that helps explain how heart disease develops. Actually, it helps explain a lot about health in general.

Arthritis, aching muscles, allergies, heart disease, some cancers, Alzheimer's disease – they all have one common denominator. It's called inflammation. Discover how to subtract it from your health equation.

Inflammation is supposed to be a hero, not a villain. It is your immune system's normal, quick response to a threat, such as an infection or injury. White blood cells rush to the scene of the crime and release chemicals to fight the intruder. The resulting inflammation restores order and protects you.

But sometimes these powerful immune cells overdo it, sort of like swatting a fly with a hammer. Then the inflammation – marked by redness, heat, swelling, and pain – becomes a bigger problem than the original threat.

Your immune system can also run wild and unleash its inflammatory chemicals on normal tissue. That's what happens in autoimmune disorders like rheumatoid arthritis.

Not all inflammation has noticeable symptoms. Sometimes inflammation works behind the scenes – and what you don't know may hurt you. Just because you don't notice inflammation doesn't mean it's not causing trouble. In fact, experts now believe inflammation plays a major role in heart attacks and strokes.

LDL cholesterol and inflammation form a deadly tag team to harm your arteries. When LDL cholesterol burrows into the artery walls, white blood cells flock to the site, leading to inflammation. This makes your artery walls stiffer and more prone to plaque buildup. It also makes the plaque more fragile and more likely to burst. Smoking, high blood pressure, and even germs also trigger inflammation and damage your artery walls.

As sneaky as inflammation is, it does leave some fingerprints behind – namely, C-reactive protein (CRP), which is produced in your liver whenever inflammation occurs.

Startling new research reveals that lowering the levels of C-reactive protein is just as important as lowering your cholesterol to reduce your heart attack risk.

In one study, men with high cholesterol and high CRP were five times more likely to suffer a heart attack. Another study found that women with the highest levels of CRP were seven times as likely to have a heart attack or stroke. Even if they didn't smoke, had normal cholesterol levels, and had no family history of heart disease, women with high CRP were still more likely to have a heart attack or stroke.

The scary thing is an estimated 25 million to 35 million healthy, middle-age Americans with normal cholesterol have CRP levels that put them in the danger zone.

Luckily, you can get a blood test that measures your CRP levels. For about $20, this important, but inexpensive, test can help assess your risk for sudden heart attack and stroke. Find out about it today. Just make sure you opt for the high-sensitivity CRP test, or hs-CRP, which more accurately detects CRP levels than the older, standard test.

You are at high risk if you have more than 3 milligrams of CRP per liter of blood. But you should start worrying if your CRP levels range from 1 to 3 mg/L. Levels below 1 mg/L put you at low risk.

The CRP test may not always be an accurate gauge of your heart attack risk. That's because people with other forms of inflammation, like arthritis, may have high levels of CRP but normal risk for heart disease. Ask your doctor if you would benefit from a CRP test.

If you need to bring your CRP levels down, lifestyle changes can do the trick. Losing weight, eating a healthy diet, exercising, and quitting smoking can all lower CRP levels. So can the cholesterol-lowering drugs called statins, although they don't work for everyone.

To further fight inflammation, turn to food. Omega-3 fatty acids, found in fatty fish, such as salmon, mackerel, albacore tuna, and sardines, reduce inflammation. These heart-healthy fats are also found in wheat germ, walnuts, flaxseed, and dark-green leafy vegetables. Add flavor and protection with turmeric and ginger, spices that serve as natural anti-inflammatories. On the other hand, keep your fat intake low. High-fat meals can trigger inflammation.

Save your gums, save your heart

Brushing and flossing not only help your teeth and gums – they are the two easiest things you can do to help your heart and brain. That's because the bacteria that cause gum disease can also damage your heart. The inflammation that results when your body tries to fight off the infection adds to the problem.

Chronic gum infections called periodontitis are painless, but wear away the bony sockets and ligaments that hold your teeth in place. People with this highly preventable condition have twice the risk of a heart attack and three times the risk of a stroke.

Reduce your risk simply by taking care of your mouth. Make sure to visit your dentist regularly – and brush and floss each day to cut your risk.

Strategies to determine your heart disease risk

Perhaps when you were in school, you dreaded tests. But now, you should welcome them. Thanks to a variety of important medical tests, doctors can determine your risk for heart disease.

Even if you don't pass every test with flying colors, you never really fail. You just have some homework to do – like losing weight, improving your diet, or taking the right medicine – before the next test. With the right approach, you can graduate to a life of good heart health.

You already know about the standard lipid profile, a blood test that measures your total cholesterol, as well as levels of LDL and HDL cholesterol and triglycerides. The importance of knowing these numbers — and what to do about them — cannot be overstated. In fact, the results of this test help determine your doctor's approach to treatment — and further tests.

Knowing your blood pressure is also essential. But beyond the two biggies, cholesterol and blood pressure, there are some other tests that may give you a better idea of your risk. Here's a quick look at some of them.

Electrocardiogram. Also called an ECG or EKG, this painless test is usually done during a routine physical or if your doctor suspects heart disease. Before the test, a technician attaches small metal sensors called electrodes to the skin on your chest, arms, and legs. The electrodes record the pattern of electrical signals from your heart as it contracts and relaxes during each heartbeat. The EKG monitor prints out a graph of your heart's electrical waves and pumping function.

An abnormal pattern can mean your heart is not getting enough oxygen through your coronary arteries. An EKG can also tell if you're having a heart attack, if you had one in the past, or if you have an abnormal heart rhythm.

The results of EKG testing may show heart disease is present, but not the extent and exact location of your narrowed coronary arteries. If an EKG indicates a significant problem with your heart function, you may be referred for angiography.

Exercise stress test. Sometimes blood flow to the heart is fine during rest, but not during physical activity. During an exercise stress test, an EKG monitors you while you walk on a treadmill or ride a stationary bicycle. Your heart rate, breathing, and blood pressure are also monitored during this test, which can last up to 15 minutes depending on your fitness level.

Other variations of an exercise stress test can achieve even more accurate results.

▸ In a nuclear medicine stress test, you receive an injection of a mildly radioactive substance. A special camera takes pictures to reveal how the radioactive material is distributed in your heart.

▸ A stress echocardiogram, performed before and after a standard exercise stress test, uses ultrasound waves to get a picture of the heart. Doctors can see the size and shape of the heart's chambers, their activity, and how much blood is ejected with each contraction. This test also detects blood clots, heart valve disorders, and other problems.

Angiography. This invasive but highly accurate test can pinpoint the location and extent of narrowing of the coronary arteries using the same approach as angioplasty. (For information about angioplasty, see page 28.)

A cardiologist threads a catheter through a blood vessel in the leg up near the small coronary arteries that supply oxygenated blood to the heart muscle. Then dye is injected into the coronary arteries to provide a contrast medium for imaging to see where blood flow may be restricted by narrowed arteries.

Angiography testing is not without risk. The procedure may sometimes damage the arteries or cause a heart attack. Therefore, it may be unnecessarily risky to do this test if heart disease is likely to be mild or if you are unwilling to have heart surgery or angioplasty.

If your family doctor thinks you may have a serious heart problem and definitely should consider angiography, and you agree, ask if he will refer you to a cardiologist who has a good reputation for performing angioplasty successfully. Ask the cardiologist to decide where the testing will be done. Then, you will probably be on track for having angioplasty rather than more-dangerous heart surgery if medical intervention is recommended after the test is completed.

Ask your doctor if conservative treatment with appropriate medication is a good alternative before deciding to have surgery or angioplasty. Usually, conservative treatment has the best statistical outcome, especially when coronary artery disease is not severe.

There is a huge medical industry devoted to expensive heart bypass surgery and angioplasty. The doctors and surgeons who make a comfortable living performing these surgeries and procedures believe they save lives. Nevertheless, these expensive treatments that appear to be lifesaving, in reality, may not be a good option for all but the most severely ill people.

Less common, but safer, tests can also shed some light on your heart's condition.

C-reactive protein test. Check out the previous story, "New theory about heart disease" to learn about this important test.

Fibrinogen test. Fibrinogen, a protein made by the liver, helps your blood clot. This can be good in some cases, such as when you have a cut or suffer internal bleeding. But too much fibrinogen can mean danger, because blood clots trigger heart attacks and strokes.

▶ A costly (about $100) blood test will let you know where you stand. Consider yourself at high risk if your fibrinogen levels top 460 milligrams per deciliter (mg/dL) of blood. From 300-460 mg/dL puts you at borderline risk, while a normal amount ranges from 150–299 mg/dL.

▶ To lower your fibrinogen level, quit smoking, exercise, get plenty of B vitamins, and eat foods rich in omega-3 fatty acids. Foods high in saturated fat and animal protein boost fibrinogen levels. People with diabetes, high blood pressure, obesity, and a sedentary lifestyle are likely to have high levels of this blood clotting factor.

Homocysteine test. This amino acid has been linked to heart disease, stroke, and peripheral vascular disease, or reduced blood flow to your hands and feet. Not all experts agree on the role it plays in heart disease, but several studies have shown that high homocysteine levels increase your risk for a heart attack. However, a recent study showed that lowering homocysteine did not reduce heart attack risk.

▸ A homocysteine blood test costs about $200. Levels above 14 micromoles per liter of blood put you at high risk. Anything below that is considered normal, although your risk starts to rise above 9 micromoles per liter of blood.

▸ Luckily, it's fairly easy to reduce your homocysteine levels. Just get plenty of B vitamins, from both foods and supplements. Exercise also helps. You may also want to cut back on meat, coffee, and alcohol.

Fasting insulin test. Following an eight-hour fast, this blood test measures the level of the hormone insulin in your blood. It helps determine whether you have insulin resistance, a condition that can lead to obesity, diabetes, and heart disease.

▸ For $75, you can find out whether you're at risk. If your fasting insulin levels exceed 25 micro international units per milliliter of blood, you are at high risk. Levels within the 15–25 range put you at borderline risk, while levels below 15 are considered normal.

▸ Losing weight and exercising should do wonders for your insulin levels. Aim for 7 percent weight loss and at least 30 minutes of moderate exercise five days a week.

Ferritin test. This protein helps your body store iron for making hemoglobin. The blood level of ferritin reflects the amount of iron stored in your body. Iron overload puts you at risk for heart disease, perhaps because the extra iron acts as a free radical to oxidize LDL cholesterol and make it more dangerous.

▸ At a cost of about $85, a blood test reveals your ferritin levels. But the normal range is so broad that the numbers might not mean much. Men should fall within 12–300 nanograms per millimeter (ng/mL) of blood. Women should be within a 12–150 ng/mL range. But if men creep above 200 ng/mL or women top 100 ng/mL, it could mean trouble.

▶ If your ferritin levels are too high, stay away from liver, red meat, soy products, and iron-enriched foods.

Lipoprotein(a) test. Known as Lp(a) and pronounced "el-pee little a," this little-known substance can cause big trouble. It carries only a small amount of LDL, but it helps form blood clots and helps prevent those clots from dissolving. High Lp(a) levels mean a 70-percent greater risk of developing heart disease over the next 10 years.

▶ Danger sets in with levels above 19 milligrams per deciliter (mg/dL) of blood. The 14–19 mg/dL range puts you at borderline risk, and below 14 mg/dL is normal. A test to determine your Lp(a) levels costs about $75.

▶ Unfortunately, there's not much you can do about your lipoprotein(a) levels, which are determined mostly by your genes. For instance, blacks and Hispanics have higher levels than whites. If your levels are high, that means you should work that much harder to lower your other risk factors.

Calcium heart scan. The mineral calcium is deposited in plaque that forms in your artery walls. A CT scan of the heart detects these deposits in your coronary arteries.

▶ Your calcium score tells you the amount of calcium – and, hence, plaque – in your heart scan. A score of 0 means there's no detectable plaque, a score of 100–300 indicates moderate plaque buildup, a score above 300 means major plaque buildup, and a score above 400 may require further tests to see if plaque is blocking blood flow to your heart.

▶ A calcium heart scan can be expensive, ranging from $250 to $600 and is unlikely to be covered by your medical insurance. But, coupled with other tests, it could give you priceless information about your heart.

Remember, you may not need all – or even most – of these tests. The result of one test often determines whether your doctor will recommend further tests. Ask your doctor if any of these tests are appropriate for you.

'Shocking' way to save your life

You don't always have time to call "911" when someone experiences signs of a heart attack. Some heart attacks cause the heart to suddenly stop beating – a condition called cardiac arrest.

To be prepared for cases like that, consider buying an automated external defibrillator (AED). These devices use an electric shock to restart a heart attack victim's heart. They come with instructions and are easy to use, but it's a good idea to get some training. You can never be too prepared for an emergency.

There's just one problem – you can't use a defibrillator on yourself. So if you live alone, it doesn't make much sense to buy one. But if you live with family or your family spends a lot of time at your house, a home defibrillator can be a lifesaver.

In 2004, the FDA cleared the Philips HeartStart Home Defibrillator for use. The only home defibrillator available without a prescription, it costs around $1,500. You can find it at some Sam's Clubs, or order online from drugstore.com, Walgreens.com, or Target.com.

Just because you have an AED doesn't mean you're in the clear. You must maintain it and keep it in an accessible spot. It doesn't do you any good if you don't know where it is. Just remember – always call for emergency help first.

High-tech ways to ward off a heart attack

Sometimes tests tell you what you don't want to know. Sometimes a healthy diet, lifestyle changes, and medication just aren't enough.

Sometimes you need to undergo a procedure to deal with the buildup of plaque in your arteries.

They may be your last resort, but procedures like angioplasties and coronary bypass surgeries can help ward off a heart attack. Here's what to expect from some common procedures.

Angioplasty. As in angiography, this procedure involves inserting a catheter into a small incision in your groin or arm and threading it through your arteries until it reaches the blocked coronary artery. Only this time, the tube has a deflated balloon at its tip. Your doctor will then inflate the balloon to compress the plaque and widen the artery.

Usually, a spring-like device called a stent holds the artery open. After the catheter is removed, the stent remains in place. New drug-coated stents, which slowly release medication to prevent scar tissue, lessen the risk of the artery becoming clogged again.

The whole procedure takes anywhere from 30 minutes to two hours, and you will probably need to stay overnight at the hospital to recover.

Angioplasty is usually a better option as a medical procedure than bypass surgery, not because it works better − it doesn't − but because it's far less risky, less costly, and doesn't cause cognitive dysfunction − problems with memory, judgment, or perception.

Coronary Artery Bypass Graft (CABG) or coronary bypass surgery. Imagine this − a 70-year-old woman named Mary is feeling tired and often has chest pain, or angina, during exercise. Her doctor is concerned about the condition of her heart and sends her to a hospital for tests. The tests show that two of the small coronary arteries that supply blood to her heart muscle are almost blocked. Mary is told she is in danger of having a heart attack and immediate heart bypass surgery is the only sure way to save her life. She agrees to have the operation. How can she refuse, given the danger?

The heart surgeon splits her breastbone, pries open her chest, stops her heart, and reroutes her blood circulation through a heart-lung machine. He takes other blood vessels from her body to use as grafts to bypass the narrowed sections of her coronary arteries. Mary's heart was stopped while the bypass grafts were sutured around the obstructed parts of her coronary arteries. She was placed on a heart-lung machine and transfused with some extra blood to maintain her circulation until that critical part of the surgery was completed. Hours later, the difficult operation is finally

> **angina** pain, pressure, or tightness in your chest triggered by a shortage of oxygen-rich blood to your heart muscle. Also called angina pectoris, these episodes most often strike during physical activity or times of emotional stress.

over. After a few weeks of recovery, Mary no longer has angina and feels better than she has in years. Another life saved by modern medicine! Or was it?

This isn't a fairy tale. Some people do have outcomes this good. However, this idealized success story is by no means guaranteed. Consider this:

▶ About 40 percent of those who have coronary bypass surgery experience serious permanent memory loss and cognitive dysfunction similar to Alzheimer's disease as a consequence of the surgery. One doctor has described the frequent impact of heart bypass surgery on mental function as equivalent to "aging the mind by 10 years or more." This is the dirty secret heart surgeons won't usually tell you.

▶ The risk of dying after coronary bypass surgery is generally greater than the risk among candidates for surgery who are instead treated with appropriate prescription drugs and counseled to make healthy lifestyle changes.

▶ The death rate from coronary bypass surgery is about 2 to 3 percent during hospitalization and 9 percent one year later after surgery performed in the very best hospitals. The surgical death rate may be two or three times higher than this in some hospitals, particularly where fewer operations are performed and heart surgeons are less skilled.

▶ The fatal "side effects" of surgery include kidney failure, lung failure, internal bleeding, stroke, and death from not infrequent infections, as well as heart failure.

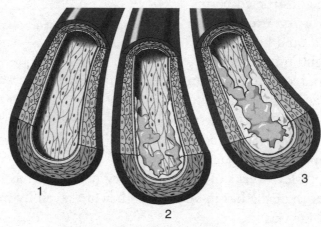

Build up of plaque in the arteries

Angioplasty or coronary bypass surgery — which is better?

Angioplasty is a less-invasive procedure than bypass surgery. A cardiologist threads a catheter through a blood vessel in the leg up into a narrowed coronary artery. He opens the artery by expanding a sturdy balloon device at the end of the catheter. An ingenious wire mesh stent, like a miniature cylindrical tomato cage, may then be clicked open to help keep the coronary artery clear.

Angioplasty may not be suitable for people who have extensive blockages in multiple coronary arteries. However, it's probably a better choice than bypass surgery for most people.

Angioplasty doesn't typically cause the serious memory loss and mental deterioration that are often a consequence of coronary bypass surgery.

Recovery from angioplasty is quick. People typically can walk out of the hospital in less than 24 hours after admission. The procedure is much less expensive than bypass surgery.

Complications are rare. In-hospital death rates are typically less than 1 percent, compared to typical fatality rates of 2 to 5 percent from bypass surgery. Survival rates after one year are better with angioplasty, but the long-term survival rates of those who survive coronary bypass surgery may be comparable to angioplasty.

One downside of angioplasty is that the procedure may need to be repeated. Restenosis, the return of a narrowing in a coronary artery, may occur in about a third of those who have angioplasty. However, the trauma from having two angioplasties is far less than the potentially deadly outcome of having a single bypass surgery.

There is less downside to angioplasty than bypass surgery if you are in the hands of a mediocre doctor or hospital team. Patients of an "A" team for heart bypass surgery might have an expected surgical death rate of 2 or 3 percent versus 5 percent or more for patients of less-skilled teams. However, with angioplasty, less-skilled doctors and their teams will probably have death rates that are still less than 1 percent.

How can you protect yourself from the medical establishment if you're a candidate for bypass surgery? First, choose a family doctor or a cardiologist who treats heart patients as conservatively as possible. Find a doctor who knows that treatment with cholesterol-lowering statin drugs and niacin and the best high blood pressure medicines, like ACE inhibitors, may be better than surgery or angioplasty. Follow the advice of a doctor who knows that healthy eating and regular exercise, like walking, can be lifesavers.

> **heart failure** the inability of the heart to pump enough blood to meet your body's needs. You may feel short of breath or have fluid build up in your lungs, legs, and abdomen. For this reason, it's also known as congestive heart failure.

Second, if your doctor recommends you have special heart tests, ask whether the tests could be done in association with a doctor or group of doctors who are skilled in performing angioplasty rather than in a hospital where patients are often referred for coronary bypass surgery after testing.

Third, if a doctor recommends bypass surgery, get a second opinion from a cardiologist in a different medical group who specializes in angioplasty. If the second opinion concurs that coronary bypass surgery is the best option, try to have the operation done in a first-class hospital by a surgeon with an excellent reputation and lots of experience.

A recent analysis of a large number of Korean heart patients treated with angioplasty versus bypass surgery showed that angioplasty definitely had better outcomes after three years. Deaths among angioplasty patients were 5.9 percent. Deaths among bypass surgery patients were 8.3 percent.

Old blood poses new threat

Out with the old and in with the new. That's the message from a recent *New England Journal of Medicine* study about the blood used in transfusions during heart surgery.

In the study, people who received blood that had been stored for more than two weeks were more likely to experience complications, including kidney failure and infection, than those who received newer blood. The people receiving stored blood also had lower short-term and long-term survival rates.

Current guidelines allow hospitals to store blood for 42 days, but that may be too long. Like milk or produce, blood has a shelf life. The longer it sits, the more it breaks down. Red blood cells become less flexible, making it harder for them to travel through narrow blood vessels and deliver much-needed oxygen to your cells.

To limit your risk, you can ask to receive fresher blood, but there's no guarantee you'll get it. In some cases, you may be able to provide some of your own blood ahead of time. Designated donations from family and friends may also work. Ask about these options when discussing your surgery with your doctor.

There is, however, a small group of people that may have better long-term survival after bypass surgery than angioplasty – the 4 percent of patients who have extensive disease in the left main coronary artery and its branches. When angiography testing finds substantial "left main" disease, cardiologists who perform angioplasty generally refer those patients to a heart surgeon if they think medical intervention is needed.

However, angiography tests that detect substantial coronary artery disease of any sort when done in hospitals where heart surgery is a big moneymaker will usually be used to justify coronary bypass surgery. Therefore, there is good reason to have such tests performed in facilities recommended by capable doctors who favor angioplasty.

Find the best hospital for heart surgery

Heart surgery, no matter how minor the procedure, is scary enough. But it's even scarier when you don't know where to have the surgery done. How do you know you're getting the best care?

You could choose one of the top 10 hospitals for heart surgery, according to *U.S. News and World Report* (see the chart on the next page). If you're at very high risk, likely to spend time in an intensive care unit, or need treatment requiring the latest technology, these big-name facilities may be your best bet.

But any hospital where many hundreds of heart surgeries are performed annually may be almost as good. Avoid hospitals and surgeons that don't have an established track record of performing hundreds of successful heart surgeries annually. These may have death rates two to five times higher than the best. It all comes down to experience. The more, the better. Ideally, you want a hospital that performs at least 450 bypass surgeries a year. Your surgeon should also do numerous procedures, preferably 125 or more each year.

Feel free to ask your surgeon questions about his experience, including number of operations, death rates, and rates of other complications. You may even be able to find such information online

33

at the Web site *healthcarechoices.org*. A little research can go a long way toward finding your best option – and much-needed peace of mind.

Hospital	City
Cleveland Clinic	Cleveland
Mayo Clinic	Rochester, Minn.
Johns Hopkins Hospital	Baltimore
Massachusetts General Hospital	Boston
Brigham and Women's Hospital	Boston
St. Luke's Episcopal Hospital-Texas Heart Institute	Houston
Duke University Medical Center	Durham, N.C.
New York-Presbyterian University Hospital of Columbia and Cornell	New York
UCLA Medical Center	Los Angeles
Barnes-Jewish Hospital/Washington University	St. Louis

Beware heart surgery side effect

People who become depressed after having coronary bypass surgery are three times more likely to experience heart failure, heart attack, or other heart problems in the first year after their surgery, one study suggests.

About 20 percent of the people who have bypass surgery become depressed while still in the hospital. If you're one of them, don't hesitate to tell your doctor. Treating your depression may save your life.

Straight talk about dangerous hospital infections

You go to the hospital to get well – not to get sick. But that's exactly what happens to many people. Approximately 2 million infections, resulting in 90,000 deaths, occur each year in United States hospitals. An additional 98,000 people die from medical errors.

You have enough to worry about when you enter a hospital for heart surgery. You certainly shouldn't have to worry about unsanitary conditions or doctors bungling your treatment.

However, infections such as methicillin-resistant *Staphylococcus aureus* (MRSA), a superbug that can't be treated with common antibiotics, and *C. difficile*, which can cause diarrhea and colitis, remain a legitimate concern. The good news is hospitals may soon be safer.

Never pay for "never events." The greatest tragedy of these infections is the loss of life. But they also cost a whopping $27 billion a year to treat.

Beginning in October 2008, Medicare will no longer pay for the cost of treating hospital-acquired infections. Nor will it cover costs related to bedsores, surgical instruments left inside patients, and several other medical errors. These types of incidents are called "never events" because they should never happen. More important, the new policy does not let hospitals pass these charges on to you, the patient.

The theory behind the new law goes like this. With hospitals solely responsible for the costs of treating infections and other medical mistakes, they will likely take significant steps to limit "never events." Otherwise, they lose money.

Do your homework. In the meantime, don't just wait for hospitals to clean up their act. Find those that already have. Do some research about area hospitals before choosing one to handle your procedure. Your computer comes in handy for this. Several Web sites post details and helpful statistics about hospitals and their safety. Here are a few of them:

▶ Hospital Compare at *www.hospitalcompare.hhs.gov*

▶ Leapfrog Group at *www.leapfroggroup.org*

▶ Agency for Healthcare Research and Quality at *www.talkingquality.gov/compendium*

▶ Health Grades at *www.healthgrades.com*

Take into account a hospital's reputation and any word-of-mouth recommendations — or warnings — from friends, relatives, or people who work there. You can also call state agencies or even contact the hospital itself to learn more about a particular facility.

Of course, you don't always have the luxury of choosing your hospital in an emergency. But doing a little homework could mean the difference between undergoing surgery at a safe, clean facility and entering a death trap.

Take matters into your own hands. No matter what hospital you enter, you can reduce your risk of trouble. The simplest way to fight infection is to wash your hands frequently — and to remind others, including visitors and hospital staff, to do the same. Here are some other steps you can take to protect yourself.

▶ Lower your weight before you undergo surgery, and you will help lower your risk of infection.

▶ Tell your family and friends not to visit if they're feeling under the weather.

Emergency care leads to more emergencies

In 2004, an ambulance rushed James Klotz to a St. Louis hospital after he suffered a heart attack. He survived the heart attack — but his troubles were just beginning.

Klotz received an IV in the ambulance and later had a pacemaker surgically implanted. Unfortunately, the procedure also left him with a dangerous MRSA infection.

He underwent 15 more operations, spent 84 days in the hospital, and lost his right leg, part of his left foot, a kidney, and most of his hearing. His wife, Mary, had to quit her job to take care of him. Recently, a jury awarded the Klotzes $2.58 million in a medical malpractice suit against the doctor and hospital.

▶ Do not shave before surgery. You may nick yourself, creating an ideal opening for germs.

▶ Watch out for surprising sources of bacteria, such as a doctor's necktie.

Bacteria can also lurk on lab coats, blood pressure cuffs, and other equipment and surfaces in a hospital. That's why hand washing can only do so much — if the rest of the hospital remains contaminated, hands won't stay clean for long.

Survival guide for leg cramp sufferers

Muscle cramps can put a kink in your routine, but that's not all. Leg pain that strikes while you walk could be a sign of intermittent claudication (IC), the second stage of peripheral artery disease (PAD).

> **intermittent claudication** a shortage of blood flow and oxygen to your legs causing muscle pain, usually while walking, that gets worse over time.

PAD results from poor circulation in your legs due to clogged arteries. Cholesterol gradually builds up inside arteries, making them harder and narrower. That means less blood can squeeze through.

You may not notice the difference until you move. Working muscles need more oxygen and nutrients than resting ones. But if your arteries are blocked, not enough blood can flow through to feed them. The result — your leg muscles starve and begin to cramp.

At first, you may feel cramps in your calves, thighs, or buttocks while walking that go away when you sit down. As PAD progresses, your muscles will cramp at rest, too. Without treatment, you can develop sores on your legs and even gangrene.

"The problem is considerable and growing," says Dr. John Farquhar, professor of Medicine and Health Research and Policy at Stanford University's School of Medicine. Christopher Gardner, his colleague and an assistant professor at Stanford's University's School of

Medicine, agrees. "Finding some treatment of benefit is of great importance to the millions who have, or will soon develop, this disorder."

You don't have to take the pain lying down. Try this advice to work past the pain of IC and PAD.

Walk more, not less. "Exercise is currently the best treatment available" for IC, say Farquhar and Gardner. Your muscles seem to use even a limited blood supply more effectively after a good workout. Not to mention, exercise is good for your cardiovascular system in general. Start small by taking a walk outside or on a treadmill.

▸ Walk until you feel pain.

▸ Stop and rest until it goes away.

▸ Start walking again.

Kerry J. Stewart, director of clinical exercise physiology at Johns Hopkins, says you should keep at it every day until you can walk for 50 minutes without stopping. Even modest goals can make a difference. "Studies show patients who exercise three or more times a week for at least three months have substantial increases in the distance they can walk without painful symptoms," says Stewart.

If you can't walk every day, try every other day – and don't give up. "Exercise should never be abandoned," urge Farquhar and Gardner.

Snuff out those cigarettes. The progression of PAD, the condition that causes IC, is directly related to how much you smoke. Quit, and you will improve both your prognosis and how far you can walk pain-free.

Control other conditions. Get a grip on high cholesterol, high blood pressure, and diabetes. These can lead to IC and make it worse. And talk with your doctor about long-term dietary changes to keep your heart and arteries healthy.

> **deep vein thrombosis** a blood clot that forms in a deep vein, usually in your leg.

Consider herbs. In recent studies, Farquhar and Gardner have found taking small, daily doses of ginkgo biloba may help open up, or dilate, some of the smaller arteries in your legs, improving circulation and easing pain. Here's their prescription for using this herb safely.

▶ Take 60 milligrams (mg) of ginkgo extract three times a day for intermittent claudication. It may take four to six months to see an improvement.

▶ If it helps, stay on it for at least a few years. During that time, your body may build new blood vessels in your legs, increasing circulation. In that case, you may be able to taper your ginkgo dose after a few years, and maybe even stop using it.

▶ Look for the brand Ginkgold made by Nature's Way. At the moment, this is the only one Farquhar and Gardner recommend because they don't believe any other brand can make the claim to be EGb 761, the ginkgo extract used in most clinical trials.

Smart tips for taking ginkgo

Ginkgo is considered a safe supplement with few side effects. Still, you need to heed a few precautions.

▶ The herb thins your blood, so avoid it if you are already on blood-thinning medications, such as aspirin or warfarin.

▶ Stop taking it at least 36 hours before undergoing surgery.

▶ Use it only under your doctor's supervision. She can help you watch for side effects and decide when to increase or decrease your dosage.

Finally, don't expect this herb to cure you. It may improve intermittent claudication (IC) symptoms, but exercise is key to a full recovery.

Triumph over congestive heart failure

You've heard the old saying "if at first you don't succeed, try, try again." When you have congestive heart failure, your weakened heart may keep trying, but it just can't pump enough blood to the rest of your body.

A healthy heart pumps at least 50 percent of the blood it receives in one beat, while a failing heart can manage only 40 percent or less. This leads to a dangerous double whammy. Not only does your body not get the blood it needs, but excess fluid can also build up in your lungs and other parts of your body.

Fluid in your lungs is called "congestion," the term that gives congestive heart failure its name. This dangerous condition can lead to disability and even death. In fact, congestive heart failure or its complications account for 20 percent of hospitalizations and almost half the deaths of people over age 65 in the United States.

Spot the signs. Often, sudden weight gain signals the first sign of congestive heart failure. The accumulation of fluid in your feet, ankles, and legs causes you to put on extra pounds. You may also feel extremely tired and out of breath when doing everyday activities, like climbing stairs, walking, or even eating.

As fluid builds up in your lungs, you may experience shortness of breath or wake up in the middle of the night with a choking feeling. To prevent that, you may have to sleep with your head propped up with several pillows rather than lying flat. You could also develop a chronic cough, which may include mucus or blood.

Consider the causes. Unlike many conditions, congestive heart failure doesn't have one easily pinpointed cause. A variety of factors could play a role in its development.

Heart failure can strike at any age, but it's much more common in people age 65 or older because your heart becomes weaker and your blood vessels become narrower as you age. Along with older people, black people and men are also more likely to have congestive heart failure.

Sometimes, specific physical defects in your heart cause the problem. Abnormal openings between the left and right chambers of your heart or a defective valve that lets blood leak back into your heart could be to blame.

High blood pressure, which makes your heart work harder, and coronary artery disease, which causes blood vessels to become narrow and clogged, can also contribute to heart failure.

Heart attacks can also lead to heart failure. After a heart attack, a section of your heart may no longer work, causing your heart to pump less. On the other hand, heart failure also increases your risk for a heart attack.

An infection or inflammation can also weaken your heart. This condition is known as cardiomyopathy. Other possible causes of heart failure include diabetes, cancer treatment, thyroid diseases, alcohol abuse, illegal drug use, and HIV/AIDS.

Treatment tips. While congestive heart failure can be deadly, fortunately, it can also be treated. It's important to work with your doctor to find a treatment plan that works for you.

In some cases, surgery can correct the problem causing your heart failure. Closing a hole between your heart's chambers, replacing a defective valve, or opening or bypassing a blocked coronary artery could do the trick. But most of the time, you can manage congestive heart failure with a combination of medication and lifestyle changes.

Drug decisions. Your doctor may try a few medications before finding the right combination or dosage. Be patient, as it could take days or weeks to notice any improvement.

▶ Vasodilators relax, or dilate, blood vessels to make it easier for your heart to pump.

▶ Diuretics help remove excess fluids and salt from your body.

▶ Digitalis helps strengthen your heartbeat, allowing your heart to pump more blood.

Each of these drugs comes with possible side effects, including dizziness, lightheadedness, skin rash, leg cramps, gout, nausea, blurred vision, confusion, fast heartbeat, and loss of appetite. Always take your medication exactly as prescribed and report any side effects immediately. For severe heart failure, you may need intravenous (IV) drugs, which can be given continuously or a few times a week.

Change for the better. Controlling congestive heart failure begins with lifestyle changes. Even if you take medication to keep your congestive heart failure under control, you still need to adopt a healthy lifestyle. Follow these 10 simple steps to control – or prevent – congestive heart failure.

▶ Cut back on salt, which causes fluids to build up in your body.

▶ Be physically active. Just make sure you stay within your limits.

▶ Lose weight if you're overweight.

▶ Eat a healthy, balanced diet rich in fiber and low in fat.

▶ Check your blood pressure regularly and keep it under control.

▶ Quit smoking.

▶ Check your cholesterol and blood sugar levels.

▶ Avoid alcohol and illegal drugs. Limit yourself to one drink per day at the most.

▶ Get enough sleep at night and rest frequently.

▶ Find ways to cope with the stress in your life. Stress hormones like cortisol and norepinephrine can have a negative impact on heart health.

5 ways to fight congestive heart failure

Congestive heart failure has a big impact on health care costs and quality of life – so every little edge you can find makes a big difference.

Some key nutrients and supplements have shown promise in the battle against heart failure. Here's a quick look at them.

▶ Coenzyme Q10. Commonly known as CoQ10, this popular vitamin-like supplement may help improve symptoms of congestive heart failure. Besides having antioxidant powers, CoQ10 may strengthen your heartbeat to boost output. It also works in the mitochondria, your cells' power sources, to improve energy production in your heart tissue.

One study found that CoQ10 treatment improved left ventricular function in people with congestive heart failure. Remember, your left ventricle pumps blood to the rest of your body.

A recent meta-analysis, or examination of several studies, found that CoQ10 helped boost ejection fraction, or the percentage of blood pumped in one beat. However, it was less effective in more severe cases of heart failure and when used with other drug treatments.

> **arrhythmia** the medical term for an abnormal heart rhythm.

Other studies found no benefit for CoQ10 treatment, but proponents for the supplement suggest these studies are flawed because the dosage tested was too small. Future studies should shed more light on the role of CoQ10 in treating heart failure.

▶ Fish oil. Omega-3 fatty acids, like those found in fatty fish, have many benefits for your heart. If you have congestive heart failure, they may be especially helpful. Fish oil fights inflammation and improves body weight in people with advanced heart failure. It may also prevent sudden death in people with heart failure by blocking the triggering of arrhythmia, or an irregular heartbeat.

▶ Resveratrol. Found in grapes and red wine, this polyphenol – or plant chemical – has several heart-healthy properties. A blocked coronary artery can reduce the blood supply to the heart muscle, leading to heart failure. In one recent study, resveratrol helped spur the growth of new blood vessels in rats three weeks after a heart attack. These new vessels help keep blood flowing to the heart in spite of a blocked artery. Resveratrol also improved the rats' left ventricular function, which is key to pumping blood to the rest of the body.

▶ Vitamins. You already know it's important to get enough vitamins, but some may be even more important when it comes to fighting heart failure.

For instance, vitamin D reduces inflammation in people with congestive heart failure. That's important because inflammation can tax your heart, forcing it to work harder to pump blood.

Vitamin C improves flow-dependent dilation, making it easier for blood to travel through your blood vessels. As an antioxidant, vitamin C works by protecting nitric oxide, which relaxes and dilates your blood vessels, from damaging free radicals.

Yet, not all vitamins help. One large study found that vitamin E offers no help for congestive heart failure. In fact, taking vitamin E supplements may even increase your risk for heart failure if you have diabetes or heart disease.

▶ Curcumin. This polyphenol, found in the curry spice turmeric, may help prevent or reverse heart enlargement, a precursor to heart failure. Animal and lab studies show curcumin counteracted the thickening and scarring of the heart muscle, as well as inflammation. It also worked in rats with high blood pressure and those who had undergone a heart attack. Adding some turmeric to your cooking could spice up your food and spruce up your defense against heart failure.

Simple 'maneuvers' calm a racing heart

Ask your doctor about vagal maneuvers. These simple exercises can slow down or stop certain types of arrhythmias, such as supraventricular tachycardia. They affect the vagus nerve, which helps control your heart rate. Your doctor might suggest you try one or more of the following self-help remedies:

▸ dunk your face in ice-cold water

▸ hold your breath while bearing down

▸ put your fingers on your eyelids and press gently

▸ cough or gag

Help your heart keep the beat

Your heart usually beats steady as a clock, but every once in a while, you may feel a quick fluttering, or your heart may suddenly speed up or slow down for no reason. This is called arrhythmia or irregular heartbeat.

Most of the time, it's nothing to worry about. However, people over the age of 60 are more likely to experience serious arrhythmias, due to heart disease, medications, and other health problems.

When your heart beats too slowly, it is called bradycardia. With this condition, your heart may slow down too much and stop beating. It may be a symptom of an underlying disease, or it could mean your heart medication, such as a beta blocker, is slowing your heartbeat too much.

When your heartbeat is too fast, it's called tachycardia. This can be caused by stress, too much caffeine, or certain types of medication, especially diet pills. While everyone's heartbeat speeds up occasionally, if you have episodes of tachycardia often, or if the episodes last longer than a few minutes, see your doctor. If your tachycardia continues for an extended time, it could lead to heart failure or a heart attack.

On the other hand, having a heart attack, heart failure, high blood pressure, diabetes, or sleep apnea can strain or weaken your heart and make you more likely to experience an arrhythmia. For this reason, you should see your doctor if you notice the signs of an irregular heartbeat.

- ▶ palpitations
- ▶ weakness
- ▶ feeling faint
- ▶ sweating
- ▶ slow or fast heartbeat
- ▶ dizziness
- ▶ anxiety
- ▶ shortness of breath or chest pain

If you have an irregular heartbeat, your doctor might prescribe medicine to help, but here are some other things you can do.

Exercise more. Regular exercise is the best way to prevent arrhythmias. The healthier and stronger your heart is, the better it can maintain its own rhythm. Check with your doctor to see what kind of exercise she recommends for you.

Stress less. If you have a problem with arrhythmia, it's even more important for you to find ways to deal with stress, since studies suggest stress might trigger dangerous arrhythmias.

Quit smoking. Aside from its other health risks, smoking makes your heart beat faster and your blood vessels narrow. This could make smoking a big contributor to tachycardia.

Dodge diet pills. The amphetamines and other stimulants in many diet pills, whether prescription or over-the-counter, can trigger tachycardia. A slow, steady weight-loss program is a better approach to solving a weight problem.

Avoid alcohol. Recent studies suggest drinking alcohol, even in moderate amounts, can worsen an irregular heartbeat.

Lay off the coffee. Caffeine jogs your heart and can cause palpitations and tachycardia. Stay away from caffeinated beverages like coffee, tea, and colas if you tend to have a rapid heartbeat.

Dodge drug interactions. Tell your doctor about any drugs you are taking, including over-the-counter drugs, when she prescribes a new one. Drug interactions can cause arrhythmias. And learn to read labels carefully. Some ingredients in cold and cough medicines may cause an irregular heartbeat.

Treat heart disease. It's an underlying cause of some arrhythmias. In these cases, consider the arrhythmia a warning sign of a much more dangerous condition, and start taking special care of your heart.

Cut your risk of 'sudden death'

The American Heart Association reports that heart disease causes 340,000 sudden deaths every year. Most of these deaths are caused by arrhythmia.

One common type of arrhythmia, called atrial fibrillation, happens when the heart's two upper chambers, the atria, beat chaotically and out of sync with the lower chambers. This leads to poor blood flow, shortness of breath, and weakness. It also increases your risk of stroke. Ventricular fibrillation is even more dangerous and often results in sudden death.

Omega-3 fatty acids may help prevent sudden death during the first hour after a heart attack. But don't wait until you have a heart attack to get more omega-3 fatty acids. You'll find two types — eicosapentaenoic acid (EPA) and docosahexaenoic acid (DHA) — in cold water fish, like salmon, mackerel, herring, and canned light tuna.

You don't have to be a fish lover to reap the protective benefits, either. Some research suggests landlubber foods, like walnuts, wheat germ, and flaxseed, as well as flaxseed oil and canola oil, might also prevent dangerous arrhythmias. These foods provide another type of omega 3 — alpha-linolenic acid (ALA).

A Danish study found a potential anti-arrhythmic effect for ALA in women. There was a link between the ALA in fat tissue and the beat-to-beat changes in heart rate, called heart rate variability. Reduced heart rate variability can lead to an irregular heartbeat and sudden death.

Another study of more than 76,000 women found that those who got the most ALA in their diet had a 38 to 40 percent lower risk of sudden death than those who got the least. In fact, every 0.1 percent increase in calories consumed from ALA led to a 12-percent reduction in sudden death.

Arrhythmia can end your life in an instant. Luckily, adding more omega-3, either from fish or plant sources, can help keep your heart beating right on time.

Work to keep your heart working

Your heart has a tough job pumping blood throughout your body. It also has a tough time avoiding danger. High cholesterol, high blood pressure, obesity, and inflammation can lead to heart attack, stroke, and other serious complications.

Your job is to keep your heart safe. A healthy diet and lifestyle can go a long way toward protecting your heart. Your doctor can also help with tests, medication, and even surgery when necessary.

Take your job seriously so your heart can keep doing its job. Because when your heart is out of work, you're out of luck.

Prescription drugs
The good and the bad

ACE heart health and strengthen blood vessels

ACE inhibitors, a category of blood pressure reducers, have been around since the 1980s. Yet, little was known about how they work until recently. New research is shedding light on how these remarkable drugs do their job. Amazingly, ACE (angiotensin-converting enzyme) inhibitors don't just reduce your blood pressure. They also improve the health of your arteries.

How they work. ACE inhibitors are prescription drugs that block angiotensin II, a powerful enzyme that narrows blood vessels. They help blood vessel walls relax, which lowers your blood pressure and allows more blood and oxygen to reach your heart. But there's more.

While it's normal for blood vessel cells to die, high blood pressure causes the cells to die faster than they can be replaced by new cells — from 1.3 percent every 30 minutes in a healthy person to 7.8 percent every 30 minutes in someone who has high blood pressure. This increase results in scarring and plaque buildup in the arteries. That's where ACE inhibitors come in.

What the studies say. Two important studies have confirmed the wonder drug status of ACE inhibitors. The most recent, nicknamed EUROPA, involved 20,000 participants and focused on the ACE inhibitor perindopril's ability to prevent heart attacks, as well as reduce plaque buildup.

The other, HOPE, is a five-year study that followed 9,000 people taking ramipril, another ACE inhibitor. All 9,000 study participants had heart disease, diabetes, or had suffered a stroke. They also had at least one other risk factor for heart disease, like high blood pressure, high cholesterol levels, or smoking.

Both studies demonstrated the remarkable ability of ACE inhibitors to do their job — and more. HOPE researchers found that the ACE inhibitor they studied not only lowered blood pressure, it reduced the risk of heart attack and diabetes.

Surprisingly, the people who took it were 30 percent less likely to develop diabetes and far less likely to have heart attacks – 150 fewer for every 1,000 people treated over a four-year period.

In a spinoff of the EUROPA study, researchers discovered something interesting. Participants with heart disease who took an ACE inhibitor saw the death rate of cells lining their arteries plummet from 7.3 percent to 4.7 percent at the end of the study. That translates to a major improvement in the health of artery walls, making them more resistant to plaque.

ACE inhibitors are well tolerated and have no ill effects on sexual desire or performance. Some users actually report they improve their mood. What's more, they're also being prescribed for diabetes-related kidney problems, and a recent study suggests ACE inhibitors are less likely to lead to diabetes than most other blood pressure drugs.

Check your blood pressure at home

Do-it-yourself monitoring may be more convenient, less costly, and even more accurate than standard approaches. It also makes you more likely to keep your blood pressure under control.

You can buy an aneroid monitor, which comes with a cuff, bulb, dial gauge, and stethoscope, for about $25. If you have hearing or vision problems or arthritis, you may prefer an electronic monitor. These range from $35 to $125, come with a cuff that automatically inflates or deflates and a digital screen, making them easier to use. Choose an arm monitor rather than a wrist or fingertip model for a more accurate reading.

To determine your blood pressure, sit quietly for five minutes and then average the results of two or more readings, taken at least a minute apart. Remember to get your blood pressure checked by a doctor at least once a year, even if you are monitoring it at home.

Information you need to know. Store your ACE inhibitors away from direct light and heat. And keep them away from damp places, like kitchen sinks and bathrooms.

If you are taking ACE inhibitors to control high blood pressure, don't use over-the-counter drugs for appetite control, colds, or congestion without first checking with your doctor. Many of these remedies tend to raise blood pressure.

Two infrequent side effects of ACE inhibitors are headaches and dry cough. Usually, the headaches can be tamed with cold packs, a hot shower, controlled breathing, or regular exercise.

It's possible to have a severe reaction to ACE inhibitors even several years after beginning treatment. So make sure you report any strange reactions − even a mild one, such as tongue swelling that goes away on its own − to your doctor immediately. As with all prescription drugs, follow your doctor's and pharmacist's instructions carefully.

The safest choice. While all prescription drugs carry some risk, ACE inhibitors are usually a much better choice than older blood pressure drugs, including calcium channel blockers, beta blockers, and thiazide diuretics.

The short-acting forms of calcium channel blockers have been linked to an increase in heart attacks and sudden death in people with unstable angina. They're also dangerous for those with heart failure, and they may impair your kidney function.

Beta blockers come with a 22-percent increased risk of diabetes and a 15-percent greater risk of stroke. Propranolol, an older beta blocker, can narrow bronchial airways and should not be used by people with asthma, emphysema, or chronic bronchitis. Side effects of beta blockers include fatigue, nightmares, depression, memory loss, and dizziness. They can also lower good HDL cholesterol. However, beta blockers do have appropriate use in certain cases such as when there is a very serious risk of heart attack with partial blockage of the left main coronary artery and its branches and in treatment of heart attack victims.

Thiazide diuretics are the blood pressure drugs most associated with diabetes. That's because they impair insulin secretion and increase insulin resistance. Like beta blockers, they may also contribute to erectile dysfunction, or impotence. Many doctors think thiazide diuretics are not the best first choice for managing high blood pressure, although they may be helpful in cases of severe fluid retention.

If you can't tolerate ACE inhibitors, one good alternative may be an angiotensin II receptor blocker (ARB). These drugs have fewer side effects, but they may not be as effective as ACE inhibitors.

Escape a dangerous potassium overload

Pay attention to potassium. ACE inhibitors can boost the level of potassium in your blood. Potassium can be good for your heart, but too much in your blood can be fatal — and this high blood pressure medicine can make it skyrocket. Use caution when taking ACE inhibitors, especially if you're also taking potassium supplements or those diuretics (water pills) that are "potassium sparing." Don't take potassium supplements or eat a lot of potassium-rich foods while taking these drugs.

Slash bad cholesterol with statins

Statins are a class of related drugs that generally do much more good than harm when used appropriately to lower high cholesterol. Niacin prescribed as timed-release Niaspan is also beneficial, and a new formulation of a statin drug combined with niacin, known as NER/S, looks especially promising because statins generally lower "bad" LDL cholesterol and niacin generally raises "good" HDL cholesterol. Beware older types of cholesterol lowering drugs such as fenofibrate (Lofibra, TriCor) and gemfibrozil (Lopid), that work by a different mechanism. These may do more harm than good.

Beating high cholesterol can be tough, but the newest statin drugs lower cholesterol levels even better. "Statin drugs will help to lower cholesterol when diet and exercise are not working well enough," explains Mindi Miller, a clinical pharmacist at Emory Healthcare and clinical assistant professor at the University of Georgia College of Pharmacy. You even have six to choose from.

▸ lovastatin (Mevacor)

▸ pravastatin (Pravachol)

▸ fluvastatin (Lescol)

▸ simvastatin (Zocor)

▸ atorvastatin (Lipitor)

▸ rosuvastatin (Crestor)

Consider the pros and cons. All the statins block a key substance your liver needs to make cholesterol. "These drugs also help to remove LDL, or bad cholesterol, from the body and can lower triglycerides," Miller says.

According to the National Heart, Lung, and Blood Institute (NHLBI), studies have reported that people who take statins end up with LDL cholesterol levels that are 20 to 60 percent lower. In addition, a statin might even boost your HDL cholesterol a little. And that's good news because HDL cholesterol helps sweep out LDL.

Two statins may give you more mileage per milligram. Before Crestor came along, research suggested that Lipitor might be the most powerful statin for cutting cholesterol. But after a six-week study of over 2,000 people with high LDL cholesterol, scientists found that Crestor reduced cholesterol more than three other statins – Lipitor,

Zocor, and Pravachol. Crestor lowered LDL by 8 percent more than Lipitor and beat the other statins by an even bigger margin.

However, one study found that Crestor might be more likely to cause dangerous muscle and kidney side effects than other statins. So talk with your doctor to determine which statin is the right choice for you.

Boost effectiveness and stay safe. Get more out of your statin and help avoid problems with these tips from Miller.

▶ Avoid grapefruit juice and bypass alcohol.

▶ Stick with a low-cholesterol, low-fat diet and keep exercising.

▶ Take the statin with a full glass of water at the same time every day.

▶ Take your statin two hours before or after antacids, like Mylanta or Maalox.

▶ Take the statin one hour before or four hours after other cholesterol medicines, like cholestyramine (Questran, Locholest, or Prevalite), colestipol (Colestid), clofibrate (Atromid-S), and fenofibrate (Tricor).

In addition, follow all directions given by your doctor and pharmacist. And talk with your doctor about getting liver function tests periodically while taking statins.

"Statins are well-tolerated by most people," says Miller. But a few of their side effects may be dangerous. Call your doctor right away if you have breathing difficulty, blurred vision, or swelling of the face, tongue, or lips.

"Report any muscle pain, tenderness, or weakness, and if you feel different in any way after starting the medication," Miller says, "call your physician immediately." These could be signs of something called statin myopathy — a condition that could lead to kidney damage and other serious problems.

Other side effects may include liver damage and memory loss. There have also been reports of people experiencing nightmares while taking statins. Reducing cholesterol means the body has less of this main building block available for making its steroid hormones, including estrogen and testosterone. Some statin users report lower sex drive while taking them.

If you have concerns about the way statins are affecting you, talk to your doctor. You can also report your experience to the Statin Effects Survey site at *www.statineffects.com*. All information submitted is confidential, but you will need to register with the site to participate and a few who participate may be contacted for additional details. They can also interact with other drugs, so make sure your doctor knows what other medication you're taking.

With higher doses come higher risks. To be safe, take only the smallest dose necessary to bring your cholesterol level down to where it should be.

Reverse heart disease, too. If you're worried that your statin isn't working, remember this. Several studies have shown that statins not only help prevent heart disease they might even reverse some of its progress if you already have it.

"Cardiologists have gone into coronary arteries of patients taking statins and actually documented that fatty buildup has diminished," says Miller. "People will not actually feel different taking statins and may still have chest pain and other symptoms, but rest assured that the medication is working."

2 easy ways to save on statin drugs

You could be just days away from paying less for your statin. Here's how you can keep more money in your wallet.

Split the cost. If you take atorvastatin (Lipitor) or pravastatin (Pravachol), you could save up to 50 percent. The secret is pill splitting. You can buy twice the dosage you need for a few cents more, then split the pill in half for two cheaper doses. But be careful. Some people have experienced dangerous effects and overdoses from splitting the wrong pill or splitting improperly. It's important to know how to do it safely.

First of all, never use a knife. Research suggests you could swallow up to 20 percent more or less medicine than you need if a pill does not break perfectly in half. Low-cost drugstore pill splitters are your best option. Talk to your doctor to find out if this strategy is best for you. If she agrees, she'll write a prescription for the high-dose statin. Talk to your doctor before you try splitting any other prescription pills, too. Splitting some kinds of pills could endanger your life.

Buy the same drug for less. Another way to save on statins is to buy generic. Simvastatin, the generic version of Zocor, pravastatin (generic Pravachol), and lovastatin (generic Mevacor) give you three, low-cost options. Generic statins contain the same active ingredients as the brand-name drugs – at a fraction of the cost. Expect to cut your costs by one-third to one-half by switching to generics. If your health insurance covers your medication, you should still save with lower co-payments.

Cleaner arteries in just 5 weeks

A new artificial HDL cholesterol may help shave buildup off artery walls. In a small study, those who got weekly intravenous infusions of this HDL had 4 percent less plaque in their arteries after just five weeks. Additional research will determine whether it's safe and effective for everyone. Stay tuned.

Statins – not just for heart health

Statins show promise for more than just heart-related problems. They may also fight Alzheimer's disease. Recent evidence comes from a University of Washington study that examined the brains of 110 people who died between the ages of 65 and 79.

People who had taken statins had significantly fewer neuro-fibrillary tangles, protein deposits in the brain that signal Alzheimer's disease. Overall, statin users cut their risk of developing Alzheimer's by 80 percent. Another study showed simvastatin (brand name Zocor), the only fat-soluble statin, was significantly effective at preventing Alzheimer's, but a water-soluble statin was not. More research is needed, but these studies suggest preventing Alzheimer's is a possible benefit of taking statins, especially simvastatin.

Statins may also lower your risk for cataracts, battle the hepatitis C virus, help with erectile dysfunction, and fight rheumatoid arthritis and cancer. Scientists are working hard to find out just how much statins can really do.

Know your alternatives

Statins may be the most powerful and famous of the cholesterol-lowering drugs, but some people, like those with liver disorders, cannot take them. Others can't tolerate their side effects. And some people need more than one drug to battle their cholesterol. Here's what else is out there.

▶ Bile acid sequestrants can reduce LDL cholesterol by 15 to 25 percent and can be combined with any other cholesterol-lowering drug. However, they may lower "good" HDL cholesterol, too. This family of drugs includes cholestyramine (Questran), colestipol (Colestid), and colesevelam (WelChol).

▶ Nicotinic acid (niacin), available as Niacor, Niaspan, or Slo Niacin, is the most effective way to raise HDL levels. It also lowers cholesterol and triglycerides. Skin flushing and itching may occur about 30 minutes after taking the drug. Taking an aspirin 30 minutes before taking niacin can help reduce these side effects.

The manufacturers of Slo Niacin claim it's clinically proven to raise HDL levels. Some experts think this polygel controlled-release niacin is superior to other over-the-counter niacin timed-release formulations.

Taking niacin may help open up clogged arteries in the legs. Niacin, as the prescription drug Niaspan, is a proven and effective treatment for coronary heart disease. Taking it hasn't been approved for peripheral artery disease (PAD), but there are anecdotal reports of benefit in related conditions. Some people report niacin has been helpful in cases of Raynaud's disease. This condition causes arteries supplying blood to your skin to narrow, decreasing blood circulation to certain areas, like fingers, toes, ears, and the tip of your nose, making them feel cold and numb.

"Flush free" over-the counter formulations of niacin aren't effective, but nonprescription regular niacin may work about as well as the more expensive drug Niaspan. If your doctor agrees, four capsules of Rexall Time Release Niacin 250 milligrams (mg), available at Walmart, taken at bedtime might have a similar effect to 1000 mg of Niaspan. But, of course, the prescription drug is the only formulation that is proven to the FDA.

▶ Fibrates, such as fenofibrate (Lofibra, Tricor) and gemfibrozil (Lopid), lower triglycerides and boost HDL levels. But total and LDL cholesterol may go up. Long-term use may also lead to gallstones. The harmful side effects of these drugs, such as increased death rates from all causes, make their use to lower cholesterol very questionable.

▶ The cholesterol absorption blocker ezetimibe (Zetia) lowers LDL by 18 percent. It's also available in the drug Vytorin, which combines ezetimibe with simvastatin, for more potent anti-cholesterol action.

Get the real story on aspirin

Discover what the pharmaceutical companies don't want you to hear. Good old-fashioned aspirin may well be the most cost-efficient way to prevent heart disease, but it pays to know who truly benefits from aspirin and who should never try it.

Salicylic acid, the main ingredient in aspirin, keeps blood cells from clumping together and sticking to the walls of your arteries. This reduces your risk of developing blood clots that can cause heart attacks and strokes.

Find out if you're a good candidate. Aspirin works differently for men and women. Recent studies show that daily aspirin therapy helps men prevent heart attacks and women prevent ischemic strokes, but not vice versa. Another large study found that aspirin might help prevent heart attacks in women over age 65. Younger women, perhaps because of the protection of estrogen, did not benefit from aspirin.

Your doctor may recommend aspirin if you're at risk for heart disease or if you've already had a heart attack. In fact, researchers recently discovered that taking aspirin before and after bypass surgery could save 8,000 lives a year in the United States.

But if you're perfectly healthy, you may be doing more harm than good. Because aspirin works as a blood thinner to keep your blood from clumping and clotting, it boosts your risk for major bleeding, ulcers, and kidney failure.

Understand the stroke connection. A stroke strikes someone every minute. That means a blood vessel becomes blocked (ischemic) or bursts (hemorrhagic), cutting off blood flow to part of the brain. Without the oxygen in blood, your brain cells die. Depending on which part of your brain is affected, you could be paralyzed on one side of your body, lose feeling, balance, bladder control, or sight or have trouble swallowing, talking, or remembering things — or a stroke can kill you.

Luckily, aspirin can improve your chances of avoiding ischemic stroke, the most common kind. In fact, several clinical trials have proven aspirin's effectiveness. A review of more than 100 studies determined that aspirin slashes the risk of future strokes by 25 to 30 percent in people who have had a minor stroke or a transient ischemic attack (TIA) But right now, experts do not advise healthy people over age 50 who have not had a stroke or TIA to take aspirin as a preventive measure. Here are some reasons why.

▶ Aspirin therapy may not work for everyone. Some people are resistant to aspirin. A recent study found that these people were three times as likely to have a stroke or heart attack or die as those who respond to aspirin.

▶ Aspirin might raise your risk for hemorrhagic stroke, the rarer kind caused by a burst blood vessel in or around your brain because of the increased risk of bleeding.

▶ Aspirin therapy comes with some drawbacks. Common side effects include stomach pain, heartburn, indigestion, nausea, and vomiting. You also run the risk of more serious side effects, such as peptic ulcers and gastrointestinal bleeding.

Talk it over with your doctor. Aspirin can interact with other drugs. Your doctor can help you determine whether aspirin is right for you. Be sure to let him know which medications, including vitamins, supplements, and herbs, you are taking. If your doctor recommends aspirin therapy, follow his instructions carefully.

If you have high blood pressure, get it under control before beginning aspirin therapy. Proceed with caution – or reconsider aspirin therapy – if you take other NSAIDs, particularly ibuprofen, or anticoagulant drugs. The combination can limit the protective effects of aspirin or increase the risk of serious side effects.

Just one tablet of aspirin a day, ranging from 81 mg to 325 mg, should give you the protection you need. If aspirin doesn't work for you, antiplatelet drugs, such as ticlopidine or clopidogrel, or anticoagulant medication might be better options. Exercising regularly, losing weight, quitting smoking, and eating a healthy diet low in fat and salt and high in fruits, vegetables, and whole grains will also help.

Block a second stroke

Aspirin can lower your risk of a second stroke by 25 percent. Ask your doctor if you should use it and how to take it.

Avoid a prescription for disaster

More than 200,000 people die each year because of medication-related problems, like drug interactions, and another 2 million are seriously injured. Fortunately, just a few minutes of reading these savvy tips could be all it takes to protect you.

Steer clear of dangerous combinations. When you take multiple medications, you multiply your risk of drug interactions. Sometimes, taking two drugs that have similar abilities can lead to big problems. At other times, one drug might change how your body absorbs, distributes, metabolizes, or excretes another drug.

Take warfarin, for example. Although many medications should not be taken with warfarin, you might be surprised to learn that the acid reducer cimetidine (Tagamet) is one of them. Cimetidine increases the effects of warfarin and could cause life-threatening bleeding. Aspirin, acetaminophen, and gemfibrozil (Lopid) are just a few of the other drugs that can cause the same problem.

And that's only the beginning. Statins don't always play well with other drugs either. For instance, if you take antibiotics like erythromycin or clarithromycin with a cholesterol-busting statin like simvastatin (Zocor,) lovastatin (Mevacor,) fluvastatin (Lescol,) and atorvastatin (Lipitor,) you could raise the amount of statins in your bloodstream. That raises your risk of a dangerous side effect that damages your muscles, threatens your kidneys, and may lead to other serious health problems. These are just two examples of these kinds of drug interactions, but that's not all.

Dodge damage from diluted drugs. You can also be at risk if you take two drugs that counteract one another. This could make one or both drugs less effective. For example, if you were to take warfarin with drugs like cholestyramine, cyclosporine, or carbamazepine, the second drug would make warfarin less effective, increasing your risk of life-threatening blood clots.

And here's another good example. Nonsteroidal anti-inflammatory drugs (NSAIDs), such as ibuprofen, may blunt the effectiveness of ACE inhibitors. They may also raise your blood pressure. Play it safe and choose acetaminophen instead.

Once again, these are just two examples. Many other drugs can cancel out the effects of medication you take for high blood pressure, high cholesterol, or heart problems.

Trounce trouble before it starts. So what do you do? Start protecting yourself with these helpful tips.

▶ Let your doctor know which medications you're taking so he can help you avoid any dangerous interactions. Also tell him about any herbs, supplements, and over-the-counter medications you take because these may interact with your medication, too. If you have more than one doctor, be sure to tell each of them everything you're taking.

▶ Always read and follow label instructions carefully, and check expiration dates on over-the-counter drugs. If you do experience any side effects, contact your doctor or pharmacist right away.

▶ Write it down. To play it safe, make a list of all the prescription medicines, OTC drugs, and supplements you take. Update the list often just in case you have a health emergency. Show the list to any doctor or nurse who sees you. Also, show the list to any pharmacist who fills a prescription for you.

▶ Have all your prescriptions filled at the same pharmacy, if you can. Each one tracks the medications you have filled there and checks for potential interactions — a safety check that could save your life.

▶ Get a "brown bag" checkup. The Institute for Safe Medicine Practices suggests showing your doctor or pharmacist all medicines and supplements you take to check for interactions or other possible problems. Schedule an appointment; put your medications, vitamins, and herbs in a bag; and take them with you.

7 questions to ask your doctor about a new Rx

Your doctor wants you to take a new prescription drug. Unfortunately, that's an extra expense and extra risk to you. Thousands of people are seriously harmed by prescribed medications every year. So what do you do?

The Institute for Safe Medication Practices (ISMP) recommends you get answers to questions like these to protect yourself from drug-related dangers.

▶ What is the name of the medicine you have prescribed? Write down the name of the medicine, as well as dosage information. One study found that most prescription errors involved the wrong drug or the wrong dose. When you pick up your prescription, compare the name and instructions on the label to the ones on your prescription and the ones you write down. If they don't match, call your doctor.

▶ Why was the medication prescribed? Some doctors have bad handwriting, so make sure you know what the prescription is for. If you can't read it, your pharmacist may not be able to, either.

▶ How do I take the medicine? After the prescription is filled, read the instructions for taking the drug. If anything differs from your doctor's instructions to you, ask the pharmacist or call your doctor immediately.

▶ What are possible side effects, and what should I do if they occur? Knowing a drug's side effects can help you determine if a problem is caused by your medication or by another medical condition.

▶ What foods, herbs, nutritional supplements, or other drugs should not be taken with this medicine? Before you ask this question, mention any allergies you have, as well as herbs, supplements, or over-the-counter (OTC) drugs you take. A safe herb or OTC medicine can turn dangerous when taken with some medications.

▶ Should I avoid any specific activities while taking this medication? Some drugs have side effects that may prevent you from spending time in the sun or doing other activities.

▶ What should I do if I miss a dose? Sometimes you should make up a missed dose, but sometimes it is safer to skip it and resume your schedule at the next dose time.

Tell your doctor about any concerns you have. If a drug seems too expensive or a pill is too big to swallow, say so. A cheaper drug or an easy-to-swallow liquid may be available.

Always ask your doctor for free drug samples whenever he writes a prescription for you. It could save you hundreds of dollars by allowing you to test drive new prescriptions first. You'll discover which ones don't work or cause terrible side effects before you spend a fortune at the pharmacy.

Samples also give you time to comparison shop for the best prices. And don't feel a bit guilty for asking – drug companies want you to use these freebies. They give loads of prescription and nonprescription samples to doctors just so they can pass them along to you.

Pick up a drug bargain

Sometimes you save more on the same drug just by buying in bulk. When you go to the grocery store, the big box of detergent costs less per ounce than the small box. The same discount pricing often applies to prescription drugs.

Ask your pharmacist if it's cheaper to buy your medication in bulk and if your insurance will cover the larger quantity. If so, talk with your doctor about writing a prescription for a larger quantity.

Sometimes it's best to stick with small amounts. Don't try to buy antibiotics or controlled substances, like narcotic pain medications, in bulk. And if you are filling a prescription for the first time, get the smaller quantity just in case it doesn't work or causes serious side effects.

Get the facts about HRT and your heart

Researchers stopped a large hormone replacement therapy (HRT) study in 2002 because they were concerned about health risks. Five years into the study, they were startled to see a significant increase in heart problems and other health concerns. Their research showed:

▶ 22 percent more cardiovascular disease

▶ a 29-percent increase in heart attacks

▶ a 41-percent jump in stroke

▶ twice the rate of blood clots

▶ a 26-percent rise in breast cancer

That translates into seven to eight more heart disease or cancer cases per 10,000 HRT users each year. That may not seem like a lot, but when you look at the population as a whole, it could mean thousands more health problems over time.

As a result, the Food and Drug Administration (FDA) began advising doctors to prescribe HRT only when benefits clearly out-weigh health risks. The FDA says doctors should prescribe HRT just long enough for successful treatment — and at the lowest effec-tive dose. What's more, women should consider other treatments for vaginal dryness and osteoporosis.

Reversing the long-held notion that HRT protects against heart disease, both the FDA and American Heart Association also began warning against using hormone therapy to reduce the chances of heart problems.

But recently, a new controversy emerged after the original researchers re-analyzed their data. The scientists now suggest that HRT may not raise the risk of heart disease in women under age 60 — as long as they start taking it soon after menopause begins, instead of waiting several years. But other experts have also exam-ined the data, and they disagree with that conclusion. The study used a form of estrogen from pregnant mare's urine, called Premarin, that's probably not as safe as estradiol extracted from yams, which has a longer established record of safety. If you take HRT, begin early and use estradiol. There may be far less risk using it than with Premarin. Talk to your doctor to learn more.

Avandia controversy – what should you do?

A recent research review of 42 studies suggests that the diabetes drug Avandia (rosiglitazone) may raise your risk of heart
attack and death from heart disease. Of the 15,560 people in
the studies who took Avandia, 86 of those had heart attacks.
But, out of the 12,283 people who didn't take Avandia, only
72 had heart attacks. Similarly, 39 Avandia users died of heart
disease compared with only 22 who didn't take Avandia.

In response to these results, the FDA issued a safety alert but
did not order Avandia's maker to add more serious warnings
about heart attack risk to the drug's label. But the FDA will
require the highly serious "black box" warning about the possible risk of congestive heart failure, a different heart problem.

The FDA will continue to evaluate whether Avandia has a role
in heart attacks, so stay tuned. But meanwhile, don't stop taking Avandia without your doctor's approval because that
could be dangerous. Instead, ask her whether you should continue taking Avandia or switch to another medication.

Nutrition know-how
Take a bite out of heart disease

'Super foods' that heal your heart

Watch television or open a magazine, and you'll see plenty of advertisements for the latest cholesterol-lowering drugs. You might think popping pills is the only way to control your cholesterol. Even your doctor may preach that the only solutions to the threat of heart disease are costly medications or exhausting exercises and bland diets.

But eating right and making simple lifestyle changes can work just as well as drugs and may even help you avoid them entirely. In fact, changing your diet can prevent heart disease and stroke, as well as slash high cholesterol and blood pressure.

The fact is, right now your kitchen is full of proven remedies shown to prevent or reverse all sorts of health conditions. Throughout this chapter, you'll learn about these "super foods" just waiting for you in the produce bins, bread racks, and even freezer shelves of your local supermarket, foods that could be healing your body now and protecting you against future illness. Make these foods your new best friends and say so long to hardened arteries, heart attacks, and strokes.

19 natural ways to lower your cholesterol

By controlling your cholesterol, you decrease your risk of developing all kinds of heart-related problems, including atherosclerosis and high blood pressure. Here's what every person can do to keep those cholesterol numbers where they should be. Check out these easy, natural ways to clear cholesterol-choked arteries.

▶ Increase the overall amount of fiber in your diet. Whole grains and fresh fruits and vegetables slash cholesterol and fill you up.

▶ Make a point of eating foods filled with soluble fiber, the kind found in oatmeal, barley, beans, apples, and other fruits and vegetables. Aim for 10 to 25 grams of soluble fiber every day.

▶ Cut back on saturated fat. These fats, found in meat and dairy products, raise your cholesterol level more than anything else in your diet.

▶ Limit the amount of trans fats you eat, the kind found in foods made with hydrogenated oils, like margarine, crackers, cookies, and french fries.

▶ Cap the total fat you eat every day at no more than 20 to 35 percent of your daily calories. Less than 7 percent should come from saturated fat.

▶ Keep your cholesterol intake below 200 milligrams a day.

▶ Load up on fruits, vegetables, and whole grains, and cut back on red meat, cheese, eggs, whole milk, processed foods, and baked goods.

▶ Snack more often. Eat several small meals throughout the day instead of three large ones. This keeps hormones, like insulin, from rising and signaling your body to make cholesterol. Just don't increase your total calories.

▶ Load up on fruits and vegetables containing the antioxidant vitamins E and C – dark leafy greens and brightly colored produce.

▶ Boost your chromium intake. Sources include apples with skins, fish and other seafood, mushrooms, liver, prunes, nuts, and asparagus.

▶ Sip alcohol in moderation – if you drink. Say when after one or two drinks.

▶ Nibble on dark chocolate. According to a Penn State study, it not only reduces LDL oxidation by 8 percent, it lifts HDL levels by 4 percent.

▶ Eat more garlic. It can slash dangerous LDL cholesterol without harming your helpful HDL. It also decreases triglycerides and improves circulation. Garlic's healing powers come from its smelly sulfur compounds, but they are only released when garlic is crushed or chopped, so take the time to prepare it properly. Let crushed garlic sit for 10 minutes before cooking.

▸ Lose weight. Being overweight increases your chances of having high LDL and low HDL levels – and a whole host of health problems. To get down to a healthy weight, you must burn more calories than you take in. That means eating less and being more active.

▸ Exercise regularly. Exercise not only helps you manage your weight, it also helps boost HDL levels. Aim for at least 30 minutes of moderate activity, such as brisk walking, every day.

▸ Quit smoking. This dangerous habit lowers HDL cholesterol and plays a major role in heart disease.

▸ Reduce stress. Researchers in London recently found that stress may raise cholesterol levels. Find ways to reduce or deal with stress in your life. Stress-coping strategies include exercising regularly, listening to music, and practicing progressive muscle relaxation.

▸ Munch on walnuts. Full of omega-3 fatty acids, walnuts have been shown to lower cholesterol in several studies. Just don't go overboard. A handful a day should do the trick.

▸ Sip on grape juice. Both purple and red grape juice have been shown to lower cholesterol. That's probably because of quercetin, a flavonoid found in grape skins, which works like an antioxidant to prevent LDL cholesterol from building up on your artery walls.

Focus on fats to beat artery-clogging cholesterol

Think you can beat high cholesterol without changing your diet? Fat chance. To lower your cholesterol, you need to eat right – and that means focusing on fats. Although fats add to the enjoyment of eating by making food tender, tasty, and pleasant-smelling, eating too much fat contributes to obesity, heart disease, high blood pressure, cancer, diabetes, and other diseases. And while fats contribute to feelings of fullness after a meal, they also stimulate your appetite.

Almost all foods contain at least traces of fat. Nutritionists refer to fat as an energy-dense food. That's because 1 gram of fat packs in nine calories, while 1 gram of carbohydrate or protein has only four calories.

Pay attention to the experts' recommendation to get no more than 20 to 35 percent of your calories from fat. But don't cut your total fat to less than 15 percent of your daily calories. According to the American Heart Association, going lower can increase your triglycerides and reduce your HDL cholesterol, just the opposite of what you want.

All fats are equal when it comes to calories, but there are big differences in how the three types – saturated, polyunsaturated, and monounsaturated – affect your health. Typically, the harder a fat is at room temperature, the more saturated and harmful it is to your arteries. Here are the main types and how much you should eat of each.

Saturated fat. Nothing raises your cholesterol more than saturated fat. Most of it comes from animal sources, like meat, egg yolk, butter, and cheese, but a few tropical plant sources, including coconut, coconut oil, and palm oil are prime sources; too. Saturated fat raises bad LDL cholesterol and increases your risk of heart disease. Less than 7 percent of your daily calories should come from saturated fat.

You can reduce the amount of saturated fat you eat by choosing low-fat or fat-free dairy products and sticking to lean cuts of meat. Trimming the fat off a pork chop, for example, can lower the saturated fat from 13 grams to 4 grams.

Trans fat. During processing, manufacturers turn some of a food's unsaturated fat into saturated fat to extend shelf life or change the taste or texture of that food. Trans fatty acids are one of the byproducts. This unusual kind of super-fat raises your LDL and may lower HDL cholesterol, as well as increase your risk for heart disease and possibly cancer. It shows up in hydrogenated vegetable oils and margarines. You can find trans fats in stick margarine, vegetable shortenings, baked goods, and french fries. Carefully read the labels on food products and limit hydrogenated oils and trans fats as much as possible.

Monounsaturated fat (MUFA). This healthy fat may lower LDL cholesterol while boosting protective HDL cholesterol. It also helps prevent arthritis, high blood pressure, diabetes, and some cancers. It should make up about 10 to 15 percent of your calories. Olive oil is one of the best sources of MUFAs, as are canola oil, peanuts, and avocado.

Use them to replace some of the unhealthy saturated fats in your diet. Switch out your regular vegetable oil with canola or extra virgin olive oil when you cook. Try slices of avocado instead of cheese on a veggie sandwich. In place of cream cheese, spread a little natural peanut butter — made from 100-percent peanuts with no hydrogenated oils — on your bagel.

Polyunsaturated fat (PUFA). About 10 percent of your calories should come from PUFAs. Like MUFAs, polyunsaturated fats lower LDL cholesterol. However, they also lower HDL. There are two main types of PUFA.

▸ Omega-3 fatty acids, found mostly in fish, boast a wealth of health benefits. They not only reduce your risk of heart attack and stroke, they also help with arthritis, Alzheimer's disease, diabetes, cancer, and depression. You'll find omega-3 in fatty fish, like salmon, tuna, mackerel, herring, and sardines. You can also find some in wheat germ, walnuts, flaxseed, and dark-green leafy vegetables.

▸ Omega-6 fatty acids, found in vegetable oils like soybean, corn, safflower, and sunflower oils, are a key part of your diet. But too much omega-6 and not enough omega-3 can lead to headaches, arthritis, asthma, arrhythmia or irregular heartbeat, and more.

Some health experts believe the balance between these two is more important than how much you get of either one. This may be particularly important if you have problems with chronic pain or depression. Unfortunately, the average person gets 10 to 25 times more omega-6 than omega-3. For better health, aim for a more even balance in your diet. Lowering the ratio of omega-6 to omega-3 to somewhere closer to the 1-to-1 ratio found in more primitive diets may provide big benefits.

New twist on the Mediterranean diet

Researchers studying the heart-healthy Mediterranean diet, rich in olive oil, made an interesting discovery. In a major study, both oils were highly beneficial, but the most benefits came from using canola oil instead of olive oil. Although both oils are high in monounsaturated fatty acids, canola oil contains more omega-3 fatty acids.

Ancient oil keeps arteries clean

Eat less fat, the experts say. But you can have your fat – within reason – and lower your blood pressure, cut cholesterol, and bust up blood clots, too, if you eat like they do in Greece and southern Italy.

Greeks know how to eat. Their typical diet includes lots of fruits, vegetables, and grains – and fat. But not just any fat. Unlike the standard American diet, where most of the fat comes from animal products, the Mediterranean diet uses olive oil as its main source of fat.

Researchers think it's no coincidence that, in spite of their high-fat diet, the Greeks hardly ever develop heart disease or hardening of the arteries, called arteriosclerosis. In fact, people in Mediterranean countries live longer than people in other parts of the world and suffer from fewer chronic diseases.

Olive oil, made by pressing ripe olives, is 77-percent monounsaturated fat, the good kind that helps rather than hurts your body. Now here's what you don't get with olive oil – cholesterol, salt, or gluten. And it has very little saturated or "bad" fat that can raise cholesterol and cause all sorts of health problems.

But olive oil is not some new miracle cure. It's been around – and prized for both cooking and healing – for thousands of years. The Cretes grew rich from exporting olive oil as far back as 2475 B.C., and both the Bible and Greek mythology refer to it. Try this ancient secret for keeping your heart in tip-top shape.

Slash high blood pressure. People in an Italian study significantly lowered their blood pressure after eating a diet rich in extra-virgin olive oil for six months. They replaced some of the saturated fat, like cream, butter, and cheese, in their diets with extra-virgin olive oil.

The oil was so powerful some people were able to cut down on their blood pressure medicine or stop taking it altogether, under the guidance of their doctors. Keep in mind, this diet was also low in total and saturated fat.

Clobbers cholesterol. This flavorful oil can be a tasty weapon against high cholesterol. Monounsaturated fats are unusual because they cut down on bad cholesterol without lowering good cholesterol.

A recent Spanish study found that virgin olive oil increased LDL's resistance to oxidation, while a new Greek study determined that even the minor components of olive oil had major powers to stop LDL oxidation. Just 20 grams, or about a tablespoon and a half a day, of olive oil could help reduce your risk of heart disease.

Blasts away blood clots. Rich in monounsaturated fat and vitamin E, this tasty oil decreases your blood's stickiness so it's less likely to clot. This lowers your blood pressure and reduces your risk for stroke.

Stops stroke. Experts have known for a while that olive oil is good for your heart. Its monounsaturated fats make your blood less likely to clot, which reduces your risk of stroke. But scientists have recently discovered a new compound in olive oil called oleocanthal — a chemical similar to ibuprofen with the same ability to reduce inflammation, an important step in preventing stroke and heart disease. Now you have another reason to pour on the "Italian butter."

Unfortunately, not all olive oils are created equal. Look for the kind labeled "extra virgin." It comes from the first press of the olives and has the most health benefits.

And remember, fat is still fattening. Oils weigh in at a hefty 120 calories a tablespoon, so you'll need to cut calories somewhere else. Don't just add olive oil to your existing diet. Use it in place of other fats, like butter, vegetable oil, and margarine.

3 types of olive oil		
Type of olive oil	**Flavor**	**Use**
extra virgin	robust, fruity flavor	drizzle over salads or vegetables
virgin	mild, fruity flavor	all-purpose cooking oil
extra light	mild flavor	can replace vegetable oils

Tiny seeds fight the 'Big Three'

That's right. You can ward off heart disease, cancer, and diabetes by eating flaxseeds.

Your liver makes the cholesterol your body needs, but extra cholesterol from the food you eat can lead to dangerous artery-clogging plaque – and maybe a heart attack. But experts say you can slash your cholesterol without expensive drugs. All you need is a secret weapon to snatch extra cholesterol away from arteries before more plaque develops – a sort of natural Roto-rooter that can help keep your arteries cleaned out.

Flaxseeds may do the trick. This miracle food lowers cholesterol, high blood pressure, and your risk of heart disease. According to one study, cholesterol levels dropped significantly when people with high cholesterol ate six slices of flaxseed bread a day. And when Dr. Philippe Szapary, assistant professor of medicine at the University of

Pennsylvania School of Medicine, and a colleague reviewed studies on flaxseed and heart disease, they found more evidence that flaxseed could help reduce harmful cholesterol.

Szapary suggests that adding flaxseed to a diet low in cholesterol and saturated fat could help reduce bad LDL cholesterol by 5 to 10 percent. That may sound small, but consider this. "If we, as a people in the United States, were all able to lower our LDL cholesterol by 5 percent, we could cut the rate of heart disease and stroke by the same amount," Szapary says.

This tasty little seed even fights cancer. When you eat flaxseed, you not only protect your heart, you also guard against breast, prostate, and colon cancers.

Fiber. "I personally think fiber is the most important component based on my own research today," says Szapary. The seeds of the flax plant have tons of soluble fiber, a miracle fiber that helps protect against high blood pressure, high cholesterol, heart disease, and even obesity and cancer.

Soluble fiber helps cut damaging LDL cholesterol by nabbing bile acids. These bile acids, necessary for digestion, are made from cholesterol. And, like a good security guard, fiber escorts those bile acids right out of your body. Then the next time your body needs to make bile acids, it pulls cholesterol out of your blood. Less cholesterol in your blood means lower cholesterol readings.

Fat. "The other component is ALA – alpha-linolenic acid," says Szapary. ALA is a type of omega-3 fatty acid, and flaxseed is the best plant source of omega-3. This heart friendly fat coats your arteries like a nonstick spray, keeping your blood flowing smoothly. It helps control high blood pressure by widening your blood vessels and preventing your blood from clumping and sticking. That way, your heart doesn't have to work as hard. ALA may help thwart other causes of heart trouble, like blood clots, irregular heartbeats, and heart disease.

Omega-3s come to the rescue again. Eating too much fat, especially saturated fat, can damage the sensitive lining of your blood vessels. Your arteries become stiff and less flexible, which can raise your blood pressure. However, many health experts say if your diet is rich in EPA or eicosapentaenoic acid, an omega-3 fatty acid found in fatty fish like salmon and mackerel, eating an occasional high-fat meal might not harm your blood vessels.

What's more, research suggests switching from foods high in omega-6, like fried foods and corn oil, to foods rich in omega-3, like fish, flaxseeds, and flaxseed oil, can help you manage your weight and control blood sugar, both of which battle diabetes.

Lignans. Flaxseed also contains special plant chemicals called lignans. In fact, flaxseed is the richest source of the lignan secoisolariciresinol diglucoside, or SDG. Your stomach breaks down SDG into two substances called enterodiol and enterolactone. Because these seem to help lower cholesterol in animals, scientists suspect they might do the same for people.

You can buy flaxseeds in most health food stores and in some grocery stores. Plus, it's easy to add to your diet. Whip the ground seeds into smoothies; sprinkle them on cereal, salads, oatmeal, applesauce, or yogurt; and throw some into your batter or dough when baking. You can even bake your own flaxseed bread. Just remember — if you have any health problems, talk with your doctor before using them. And for best results, read these pointers before you start.

▶ For the most nutrition, grind the seeds with a coffee grinder and use them immediately.

▶ Flaxseed is an intense source of fiber. One tablespoon can contain up to 2.2 grams. To avoid gas and indigestion, start small and add flaxseed to your diet gradually.

▶ Stick with the whole seeds, not the oil, if your main goal is to lower your cholesterol. "Flaxseed oil doesn't have any of the fiber and none of the lignans so you're really only getting the omega-3," says Szapary. "The flaxseed capsules won't have any effect on your cholesterol."

Pour on protection

You can store flaxseed oil in the refrigerator if you plan to use it within two months, or keep it in the freezer for up to a year. Do a sniff test. If it smells overly fishy, it's probably gone bad.

Use the oil on salads and on vegetables instead of butter, but don't cook with it. It can actually break down into harmful compounds when heated.

Great reasons to eat more nuts

The evidence is piling up – nuts are good for your heart. In fact, eating more nuts can save your life. Although high in fat, they're cholesterol-free. And the fats they boast tend to be the good kind – cholesterol-lowering monounsaturated fatty acids (MUFAs), the same kind found in olive oil, and the polyunsaturated fatty acid (PUFA) known as omega-3, also found in fish oil. Scientists think omega-3 fatty acids may pitch in to avert the irregular heartbeat that can cause "sudden death" – death within an hour of a heart attack.

In addition, most nuts serve up lots of arginine, an amino acid your body uses to make a substance that fights plaque buildup in your arteries. And the folate in nuts helps keep a lid on homocysteine, another amino acid that can damage arteries if too much builds up in your blood. What's more, their stores of soluble fiber may cut LDL cholesterol, and many are good sources of heart-healthy minerals, like copper and magnesium.

Over the years, scientists have gathered lots of research on the heart-healing power of nuts.

▶ Researchers studying 30,000 Seventh Day Adventists found that those who ate nuts at least five times a week slashed heart attack risk by 50 percent, compared to those who ate them less than once a week.

▶ Pennsylvania State University experts found that eating an ounce or more of nuts five times a week could bring down your risk of heart disease up to 39 percent.

▶ A 17-year study of 21,000 male doctors suggested the odds of death from heart disease were 30 percent lower in men who ate nuts at least twice a week. Compared to those eating nuts less often, men who ate two or more 1-ounce servings of nuts weekly had 47 percent less risk of sudden death.

▶ A study of 40,000 postmenopausal women also found a lower risk of heart disease among frequent nut eaters.

Different nuts may help your heart in different ways. Small studies hint that almonds, pecans, walnuts, and macadamias may trim cholesterol. Pistachios lead all other nuts in potassium — a mineral that eases blood pressure. And peanuts — technically, they are legumes, not nuts — contain resveratrol, a plant estrogen that works like an antioxidant to combat heart disease. Here are some more tasty nuts worth nibbling.

Walnuts. Go ahead and say nuts to heart disease. Proven to lower cholesterol, walnuts are a good source of a particular omega-3 fatty acid called alpha-linolenic acid (ALA), plus they're high in the antioxidant vitamin E. One study of people living in a walnut-producing area of France linked eating lots of walnuts with an increase in good HDL cholesterol.

What's more, walnuts can thin your blood and help prevent clots, and a new study finds that these particular nutmeats actually restore flexibility to your arteries. A trial with 20 men and women showed that eating eight to 13 walnuts a day improves blood flow by making your arteries more elastic. Walnuts also increased a substance called apo A1, which is associated with a lower risk of heart disease.

Know your nuts

Nuts	Nuts per 1-ounce serving	Calories	Protein (grams)
Almonds	24	160	6
Brazils	6-8	190	4
Cashews (dry roasted)	18	160	4
Hazelnuts	20	180	4
Macadamias (dry roasted)	10–12	200	2
Peanuts	28	170	7
Pecans	20 halves	200	3
Pine nuts (pignolias)	157	190	4
Pistachios (dry roasted)	49	160	6
Walnuts	14 halves	190	4

Almonds. Ounce for ounce, almonds pack nearly as much protein as red meat. They are cholesterol-free, low in saturated fat, and high in vitamin E, calcium, and fiber. They're pretty good for your heart, too.

In one study, people who added almonds to their diets lowered their total cholesterol by 7 percent and LDL cholesterol by 10 percent. A separate clinical trial found that eating almost 4 ounces of almonds each day as part of a diet low in saturated fat cut total cholesterol levels about 20 points, or nearly 9 percent. Experts credit the drop to getting more MUFAs from almonds, while cutting back on heart-damaging saturated fats.

Fat (grams)				Omega-6 fatty acids (grams)	Omega-3 fatty acids (grams)
Total	Sat	Mono	Poly		
14	1	9	3	3	0
19	5	7	7	6.8	.02
13	3	8	2	2.2	.05
17	1.5	13	2	2.2	.02
22	3	17	.5	.4	.06
14	2	7	5	4.4	0
20	2	12	6	5.9	.28
20	2	6	10	9.4	.05
13	1.5	7	4	3.9	.07
18	1.5	2.5	13	10.8	2.6

Peanuts. This popular legume may provide a unique way to get heart-healthy MUFAs. Peanuts contain the same antioxidant found in grape skins, and this antioxidant is partly responsible for red wine's ability to lower heart disease risk.

In fact, you could lower your bad LDL cholesterol by using peanut cooking oil. One study tested five different kinds of diets – a typical American diet, a low-fat diet, an olive-oil diet, a peanut/peanut butter diet, and a peanut oil diet. The peanut diets contained small amounts of peanuts daily. The study found that the olive oil and the peanut diets, which were low in saturated fat and high in monounsaturated fat, all lowered bad LDL cholesterol. The low-fat diet lowered bad LDL cholesterol, too, but it also lowered good HDL cholesterol and raised triglyceride levels. So put some peanut oil in your pantry today. Your heart will thank you.

Ease the high-fat assault on your arteries by including a handful of nuts at mealtime. However, don't just add them to your diet. Eat nuts in place of other high-calorie foods. Otherwise, their high fat and calorie content could lead to weight gain. A review of nut research found that nut eaters don't have a higher body mass index than people who don't eat nuts — as long as the nuts replace another high-calorie food in the diet.

Studies suggest 1 to 2 ounces of nuts a day — about a handful — may be enough to do your heart good. Sample almonds, walnuts, peanuts, pecans, chestnuts, hazelnuts, pistachios, and more. Just try to avoid nuts coated with candy, sugar, honey, or salt. If you're salt-sensitive, check the label for sodium content.

Nuts are a common cause of food allergies. Call for emergency help if you experience any of these symptoms within an hour of eating nuts — skin rash, scratchy or swollen throat, stuffy or runny nose, sneezing, difficulty breathing, stomach upset, vomiting, diarrhea, or bloating.

Grab help by the handful

The Food and Drug Administration (FDA) recently approved a health claim for labels of whole or chopped walnuts. The claim says that "supportive but not conclusive research" shows that eating 1.5 ounces of walnuts daily may reduce heart disease risk — but only if the nuts don't boost calorie intake and are part of a low-cholesterol, low-saturated-fat diet.

The FDA is considering a similarly worded claim for most other nuts. But cashews, macadamias, Brazil nuts, and some pine nut varieties won't ever display the claim because they have too much saturated fat.

Fishy solution for a healthy heart

Is artery disease lurking in your veins? If you have fatty plaque buildup, a clot in your arm or leg can gridlock your arteries just like a 5 p.m. traffic jam. That situation puts you at risk for tissue damage or even a heart attack. Your doctor can do a simple test to determine if you have PAD – peripheral artery disease. She simply compares the blood pressure readings at your arm and ankle to assess your risk. Ask about it today, especially if you have leg pain. If she does find PAD, heart medicines are not your only option. You have some natural ways to control your cholesterol and thin your blood.

You know you should watch the fats in your diet, but don't go overboard. Cutting back on your fat intake too much can do your heart more harm than good. That's because your triglyceride levels can shoot up even as your good HDL cholesterol levels drop – if you try to maintain a diet with less than 15 percent fat.

The key to heart health is not to cut all the fat out of your diet. Instead, you should aim to get the right kind of fat. The omega-3 essential fatty acids in cold-water fish, like tuna, salmon, and mackerel, can bring down your LDL cholesterol numbers and keep your triglycerides under control. They will also keep your blood from getting "sticky" and clogging your arteries – both spelling health for your heart.

In fact, if you add just one 3-ounce serving of fatty fish to your diet every week, you can cut your risk of a heart attack in half. A study of people at risk for heart disease found that even people who had diabetes or who smoked got good results from eating a serving of fish every week. The fish eaters were 38 percent less likely to have a heart problem during the study than those who didn't partake.

If you've already had a heart attack, just taking a fish oil supplement can lower the threat of a second attack by 10 percent. Don't ignore the idea of omega-3 if you can't stomach seafood. You can get plenty of omega-3 fatty acids from flaxseeds and flaxseed oil or from fish oil supplements.

Buy fresher fish

Look for the following signs of freshness when buying fish.

▶ moist, slippery, and shiny skin, with bright coloring and firmly attached scales

▶ bright red gills, a fresh smell, and clear eyes that have not sunk into the surrounding skin

▶ firm flesh on whole fish, fillets, and steaks, which bounces back when pressed

▶ moist flesh on fillets and steaks, with an even white or red coloring

Fish tastes best when cooked fresh, but you can wrap it in wax paper and refrigerate it for up to two days. You can also freeze it for up to six months.

Avocados — armor for your heart

According to legend, a Mayan princess ate the first avocado in 291 B.C. Fortunately, you don't have to be royalty to reap the rewards of this tasty tropical fruit.

Nicknamed "alligator pears" because of their bumpy exteriors, avocados come in several varieties. Some have a green covering. Others are dark purple or almost black. Some are smooth, while others are bumpy. Some are small, and others weigh as much as 4 pounds. Yet, when you slice them open, they all have the same delicious light-green, nutty-flavored flesh inside.

Loaded with monounsaturated fat, potassium, fiber, and antioxidants, the avocado lowers bad and raises good cholesterol levels, plus fights high blood pressure, heart disease, and stroke. This "super fruit" has even been shown to ease arthritis, eliminate kidney stones, and aid digestion.

Tackles bad cholesterol. Eating high-fat avocados may help lower your total cholesterol without cutting "good" HDL cholesterol. According to a Mexican study, avocados might even boost your levels of HDL by 11 percent. Although the avocado is high in fat – 30 grams per fruit – it's mostly monounsaturated fat. This fat helps protect good HDL cholesterol, while wiping out the bad LDL cholesterol that clogs your arteries.

But there's more than just monounsaturated fat at work. An avocado contains a whopping 13 grams of fiber, as well as a plant chemical called beta-sitosterol. These both help lower cholesterol. Throw in vitamins C and E – powerful antioxidants that prevent dangerous free radicals from reacting with the cholesterol in your blood – and it all adds up to a healthier you.

In fact, one study from Australia demonstrated how eating half to one-and-a-half avocados a day for three weeks could lower your total cholesterol by more than 8 percent without lowering your HDL cholesterol. During the same study, a low-fat, high-carbohydrate diet also lowered the participants' total cholesterol – but slashed the "good" cholesterol by almost 14 percent.

Bashes high blood pressure. You've probably heard that bananas are a good source of potassium. What you probably don't know is that avocados, with over 1,200 milligrams of potassium per fruit, contain more than two-and-a-half times as much potassium as a banana. This is important because many studies show that potassium helps lower your blood pressure.

Magnesium, another important mineral found in avocados, could help lower your blood pressure, too. Some researchers think magnesium relaxes blood vessels and allows them to open wider. This gives blood more room to flow freely, reducing blood pressure, but results have been mixed. Some studies show magnesium lowers blood pressure, while others show no effect.

Strikes out stroke. When it comes to taking on a deadly killer like stroke, who wants to fight fair? Gang up on stroke with avocado's three heavy hitters – potassium, magnesium, and fiber.

In the Health Professionals Follow-Up Study, which included more than 43,000 men, researchers found that the men who got the most potassium in their diet were 38 percent less likely to have a stroke as those who got the least. Results were lower for fiber (30 percent) and magnesium (30 percent).

Hammers heart disease. By controlling your cholesterol and blood pressure, avocados can help reduce your risk of heart disease. This fruit can reduce the amount of triglycerides, another type of fat, in your blood. A high triglyceride level can be a warning sign of heart disease. What's more, if you increase your daily fiber intake by 10 grams – less than the amount in one avocado – you decrease your risk of heart disease by 19 percent.

Plus, avocados have more folate per ounce than any other fruit, according to the California Avocado Commission. Research has linked this B vitamin to a reduced risk of heart disease. It helps your heart by keeping homocysteine from building up to dangerous levels. Homocysteine, a by-product of protein metabolism, can harm your arteries and increase your chances of a heart attack or stroke.

Stamps out kidney stones. Avocados are excellent sources of potassium, magnesium, and vitamin B6 – three of the most important nutrients for preventing kidney stones. Both magnesium and B6 help your body control its oxalate levels, while potassium decreases the amount of calcium in your urine. Together, they can help you kick calcium oxalate kidney stones, the most common kind.

Eases arthritic joints. You can kill two diseases with one avocado stone. Those ever-helpful MUFAs in avocados seem to relieve inflammation and reduce joint swelling in people with rheumatoid arthritis, an illness also linked to heart disease. It works on RA by controlling cytokines, molecules that have to do with inflammation.

Do your digestion good. Simply eating more fiber can treat all sorts of digestive ills, from heartburn and hemorrhoids to constipation, diarrhea, and inflammatory bowel disease (IBD), not to mention prevent diverticular disease, appendicitis, gallstones, and hiatal hernias. Fiber helps add bulk and softness to stool, helping it move more smoothly through your digestive tract and toning your digestive muscles. With each avocado packing an amazing 13 grams of fiber – more than half the recommended daily amount for women and more than a third for men – what more could you ask for from one simple fruit?

Ripen avocados faster

Avocados go all the way back to the 9th century – almost as long as you've been waiting for the one on your counter to ripen. To speed up the process, seal the avocado in a plastic bag along with an apple or ripe banana. Keep the bag at room temperature until the avocado becomes soft and ripe. You'll know they're ripe when the skin is dark, and it yields to gentle pressure. You can also try burying them in a bowl of flour.

Cut LDL with a butter knife

Is there a margarine you can spread on your toast that's kind to your heart? It may sound too good to be true, but this margarine actually clobbers artery-clogging cholesterol. The secret ingredients come from two new fats. "Stanols and sterols bind with cholesterol found in food and with bile acids used to make cholesterol in the body," says Lona Sandon, assistant professor of clinical nutrition at The University of Texas Southwestern Medical Center at Dallas. This binding prevents cholesterol from being absorbed into the bloodstream, she says.

Both stanols and sterols come from plants. Sterols from soybeans are the power behind Take Control, a Lipton Foods margarine. But a stanol is the secret weapon of Benecol – the competing margarine from Johnson & Johnson subsidiary, McNeil Consumer Products Co. The stanol in canola-based Benecol is a special byproduct from the wood-processing industry.

Check the evidence. You're more likely to have heart disease if you have too much low-density lipoprotein (LDL) cholesterol. That's why LDL is nicknamed "bad" cholesterol. But stanol and sterol margarines can help.

A review of more than 40 research studies concluded that just 2 grams of stanols or sterols daily could help cut LDL cholesterol levels by about 10 percent.

Because increasing your intake to more than 2 grams a day isn't more effective, it's not recommended. However, if you combine these margarines with a low-fat diet or with medications, you might cut LDL by up to 20 percent.

But that's not all. The evidence that stanols and sterols help fight heart disease is strong, so the Food and Drug Administration authorized a labeling health claim for sterol- and stanol-powered foods. As long as the foods are low-fat and low-cholesterol, their labels can state they may help slash heart disease risk.

Although stanol and sterol margarines are generally recognized as safe, the products haven't been around long enough for long-term safety studies.

Plan your attack. Stanol and sterol margarines are most helpful if your cholesterol is only modestly high – around 200 to 239 mg/dL.

"The most benefit seems to come with about 2 grams per day of the plant stanol/sterol – or using 1 tablespoon of the spread, two to three times per day while following a healthy diet and exercise plan," says Sandon.

To get maximum mileage from your margarine, use it to replace fats you normally eat. Otherwise, you'll gain weight and cancel out the spread's benefits.

Eat colorful fruits and vegetables to help control weight and prevent nutrient losses. "These margarines may lower carotenoid levels in the blood by 10 to 20 percent," Sandon says. But you can fix that. "Just one extra serving of a carotenoid-rich fruit or vegetable — such as carrots, sweet potato, pumpkin, tomatoes, apricots, or spinach — has been shown to prevent any lowering of carotene levels," Sandon says.

Don't use these margarines to replace your cholesterol drugs. Although the spreads work well with medicines like statins, they're no substitute.

Look for cholesterol-cutting margarine in your grocery store. If you plan to use the margarine for cooking or want zero trans fats, check the labels. "Some versions of the products are trans-fat free, which means they contain less than 0.5 grams of trans fat per serving."

"The regular stanol margarines that can be used for baking and cooking contain less than 1 gram of trans fat per serving," says Sandon. "The amount of trans fat is no more, maybe even less, than one would find in a typical margarine."

Talk with your doctor before you try sterol or stanol margarines, especially if you take cyclosporine or similar drugs.

Snack on sunflower seeds

Get a boost from these tasty tidbits. They're loaded with vitamin E, a powerful antioxidant that stops LDL cholesterol — the bad kind — before it can form plaque that clogs up your arteries. Vitamin E has other anti-clotting powers, too, so it's easier for your heart to pump blood and keep your blood pressure down. It also guards against hardening of the arteries, stroke, and heart attack. Remove the tasty sunflower morsel from its shell, or buy the little seeds already shelled and ready to sprinkle on salads or munch by the handful.

Nutritional superhero to the rescue

It's a bird, it's a plane, it's … fiber! This nutritional superhero can rescue you from high cholesterol, high blood pressure, stroke, and even weight gain.

Back in the 1940s, Dr. Denis Burkitt began to notice the importance of diet to good health. Working as a surgeon in East Africa, he rarely saw conditions, like constipation, hemorrhoids, and appendicitis, that were widespread in the Western world. He came to believe the amount of fiber, or roughage, people eat could explain why.

Fiber is the part of fruits, vegetables, and grains your body can't digest. There are two kinds, both important in keeping you healthy. Ideally, you want to get a balance of both types in your diet.

▸ Soluble fiber turns soft and sticky in your body, slowing things down in your stomach and small intestine. This gives your body more time to whisk away bad cholesterol and absorb carbohydrates. Dried beans, peas, oats, barley, flaxseed, and many other fruits and vegetables contain soluble fiber.

▸ Insoluble fiber passes right through your digestive system. It keeps your bowels moving smoothly and tones your digestive muscles. It also adds bulk to your stool and speeds it through your large intestine. This guards against constipation, diverticulosis, and possibly colon cancer. Look for insoluble fiber in whole-wheat foods, bran, and fruits and veggies with tough, chewy textures.

You'll also probably want to up your fiber intake, because most people fall short of recommended levels. In his book *Eat Right − To Stay Healthy and Enjoy Life More*, published over 20 years ago, Burkitt pointed out that people in developing nations tended to eat about 60 grams (g) of fiber a day. In Western countries, the average amount was about 20 g.

Today, fiber intake is even lower. According to the National Institutes of Health, Americans eat only 5 to 20 g of fiber a day. If you are among those eating the lowest amounts, you fall far short of the recommended 20 to 35 g. Many nutritionists believe you'd be healthier with the higher amounts Burkitt recommended. According to the Institute of Medicine, men over age 50 should eat at least 30 g of fiber each day, while women the same age should aim for 21 g. Make more fiber a priority in your diet, and here's what it could help you do.

Drop high blood pressure. A four-year study found that women who ate more than 25 g of fiber a day were about 25 percent less likely to develop high blood pressure as women who ate less than 10 g of fiber every day. If you have high blood pressure, adding just 10 g of fiber to your diet every day can slash your risk of stroke a whopping 41 percent.

Slash your stroke risk. Fiber helps lower cholesterol, too. Cholesterol buildup can block blood vessels, causing an ischemic stroke. About 80 percent of all strokes fall under this category. High blood pressure increases your risk of a hemorrhagic stroke – when a blood vessel in or near your brain bursts. Because fiber can lower blood pressure and cholesterol, it can also reduce your risk of both types of stroke.

Researchers reviewed 77 different studies that looked at the effect of soluble fiber on total cholesterol, and they found significant reductions in 88 percent of them. Nearly all the studies showed results from a high-fiber diet in a matter of weeks. The source of the fiber varied in the studies from pectin (found in apples and other fruit) to psyllium (the main ingredient in Metamucil), dried beans to raw carrots.

Shed spare pounds. Why all the fuss about fiber? Well, for starters, it can help you lose weight. It has absolutely no calories, and what's more, your body needs it to function at its peak. Not only does fiber move through your system without adding calories, it also makes you feel full longer, so you're not snacking between meals. It may even block the absorption of some of the fat and protein you eat.

And because many high-fiber foods – like fruits and vegetables – are low in calories, you can actually eat more, not less, of some and still lose weight and get healthy. Along with helping you stay in shape, fiber can help prevent conditions like constipation, hemorrhoids, diverticulosis, diabetes, heart attack, stroke, and cancer.

While fiber supplements are available, your best bet is to get your fiber from foods, which also contain lots of nutrients. Fruits, vegetables, and whole-grain breads and cereals are good sources of fiber. For example, one potato with skin has 5 g of fiber, an orange has 3 g, and a cup of raisin bran has 8 g. Just make sure to add fiber to your diet gradually. Adding too much too quickly can cause gas, abdominal cramps, bloating, and diarrhea.

5 ways to fit more fiber in your day

Reaching your high-fiber goals can seem a daunting task, but these five tips make it simple.

▶ Start with cereal. Read food labels to find a whole-grain cereal that contains at least 5 grams of fiber per serving. Top it off with raisins, sliced bananas, or chopped apple.

▶ Eat raw veggies. Munch on carrot or celery sticks, and lunch on a crunchy garden salad. When you cook veggies, steam or sauté them just until tender.

▶ Snack on fresh and dried fruits. And whenever possible, eat the skins of fruits and vegetables. That's where you'll find the most fiber.

▶ Substitute brown rice for white. With that switch, you'll triple the fiber. Try some less-familiar, unprocessed grains as well, like bulgur, couscous, or kasha.

▶ Add beans to soups and stews. Replace meat a couple of times a week with dishes like bean burritos or red beans and rice.

A sweet treat that heals your heart

In the Garden of Eden, Adam and Eve used fig leaves for clothing. Fashions have changed a lot since then, but figs have never gone out of style. This sweet, take-along snack gives you a triple punch of stroke-stopping, heart-healing nutrients, antioxidants, and fiber.

These sweet fruits were mentioned in writings as far back as 3000 B.C. Cleopatra enjoyed figs, and the Roman writer Pliny the Elder praised them for their power to get rid of wrinkles. Today, you can find figs in a variety of forms, including the popular Fig Newton cookie – a healthy alternative to most desserts.

When you get down to it, figs mean fiber. Pound for pound, figs pack more of this precious stuff than any other fruit or vegetable. Five figs, fresh or dried, give you a whopping 9 grams of fiber, more than a third of the recommended amount. Besides fiber, figs are loaded with minerals and other nutrients to help fend off heart disease, cancer, constipation, and even diabetes.

Dried figs are especially good for you because they're chock full of antioxidants. They also make a sweet and portable snack. Plus, figs taste great. These chewy treats, sometimes called "inside-out strawberries," contain tiny, edible seeds. Bite into a deliciously healthy fig, and you'll feel just a little bit closer to paradise.

Cut cholesterol. "If you eat a lot of fiber, you will have a better cholesterol level," says Dr. Joe Vinson, chemistry professor at the University of Scranton in Pennsylvania and an expert on figs. The bottom line is lowering artery-clogging cholesterol lowers your risk of heart disease.

Figs also contain lots of polyphenols, plant compounds that act as antioxidants. Polyphenols stop low-density lipoprotein (LDL or "bad") cholesterol from oxidizing then building up in your arteries, and they keep your blood from becoming sticky and clumping together.

Save you from strokes. The triple punch of fiber, potassium, and magnesium in figs means extra protection from stroke, especially if you have high blood pressure. Even though fewer people are suffering from strokes these days — thanks to better treatments for high blood pressure — strokes still cause one out of every 15 deaths. Experts agree, more nutrient-rich fruits and vegetables should be your first line of defense.

Halt high blood pressure. Experts recommend figs for people with high blood pressure. Their combination of potassium and calcium, along with eating less sodium, can give your body the one-two punch it needs to put a lid on blood pressure.

Manage weight. Remember, fiber can help you lose weight, which will not only shrink your waistline but your risk of heart disease and other health problems, too. "Figs are very filling," Vinson explains, "so you'd decrease your consumption of other things if you ate more figs They're not super-high in calories or fat, either." You'll get just 48 calories and almost no fat in every dried fig.

Deal with diabetes. If you're worried about high blood sugar but still want a tasty treat, look no further than the fig.

"Figs are not a high-carbohydrate food," says Vinson, "so they would be typically a good thing for someone who has diabetes to consume. And fiber will lower your glucose." Keep in mind, fiber slows the amount of glucose your body absorbs from your small intestines.

The evidence backs Vinson up, too. A recent study found that a high-fiber diet — 50 grams per day — helped keep blood sugar, insulin, and cholesterol under control in people with diabetes.

Eating chewy, delicious figs is a tasty way to get more fiber. In fact, the American Diabetes Association offers recipes that include figs. Visit their Web site at *www.diabetes.org*.

Top 20 antioxidant foods

Researchers have measured and studied antioxidants in food at the Jean Mayer USDA Human Nutrition Research Center on Aging at Tufts University in Boston. They determined what foods have the highest Oxygen Radical Absorbance Capacity (ORAC) score. A food's ORAC score is a measure of the total amount of antioxidants in that food. Edibles with high ORAC values, like these top scorers, do the best job at helping your cells repair themselves and fight disease.

Food	Serving size	ORAC units per serving
small red bean (dried)	half cup	13727
wild blueberry	1 cup	13427
red kidney bean	half cup	13259
pinto bean	half cup	11864
blueberry (cultivated)	1 cup	9019
cranberry	1 cup (whole)	8983
artichoke (hearts, cooked)	1 cup	7904
blackberry	1 cup	7701
dried plum	half cup	7291
raspberry	1 cup	6058
strawberry	1 cup	5938
red Delicious apple	one	5900
Granny Smith apple	one	5381
pecan	1 ounce	5095
sweet cherry	1 cup	4873
black plum	one	4844
russet potato (cooked)	one	4649
black bean (dried)	half cup	4181
plum	one	4118
Gala apple	one	3903

Nutritional powerhouse great for snacking

Movie stars frequently change their ordinary, given names to something more glamorous once they're in the spotlight. That's what happened with your old friend the prune.

Ever since researchers discovered that prunes are packed with antioxidants, this dried fruit has gotten lots of attention. Who knew so much goodness was hiding inside that black, wrinkly package?

Like the star it hopes to become, the prune has changed its name and is now known as a "dried plum." But a prune by any name would taste as sweet. It would also give you lots of fiber, protect you from free radical damage, and maybe even lower your cholesterol. Dried plums are also a good source of potassium – important for a healthy heart and strong bones. And you can eat 10 sweet, chewy dried plums filled with nutrition for only 200 calories.

Clobber high cholesterol. Unless you're a horse, you can only eat so many oats. But now you can clobber cholesterol without oat bran. The alternative – dried plums. These sweet, small fruits can lower dangerous LDL cholesterol in just four weeks.

Eating a diet high in fiber can help lower your cholesterol, and a study of dried plums helped prove it. Researchers in the Department of Nutrition at the University of California, Davis, gave a group of 41 men with mildly high cholesterol 12 dried plums each day for four weeks. They then gave the same men a couple of glasses of grape juice daily for four more weeks. The men were told not to change their eating or exercise habits during the study.

Tests showed that LDL cholesterol – the kind you want to keep low – was significantly lower during the dried plum period than during the grape juice period. This is great news if your cholesterol is starting to creep upward, and you don't want to take medicine. Lower cholesterol means you're less likely to develop heart disease.

Put the brakes on aging. For years, scientists have wondered what people can do to hold on to the health and vitality of their youth. The latest thinking is that antioxidants – free radical fighters found mainly in fruits and vegetables – are the key to keeping young and avoiding cell damage.

At 7,291 ORACs (Oxygen Radical Absorbance Capacity or total amount of antioxidants in a food) per half-cup serving, it registered more than twice as many antioxidants as its little wrinkled cousin, the raisin.

When animals were given foods high in antioxidants, they showed less signs of aging on memory tests. Scientists think antioxidants may be an important key to protecting yourself from diseases of aging and even cancer. In fact, the loss of brain function in certain diseases like Parkinson's and Alzheimer's seems to be from free radical damage.

The USDA's Agricultural Research Service Administrator Floyd P. Horn has seen the future of treating age-related diseases, and it looks a lot like your grandma's vegetable garden.

"If these findings are borne out in further research," he says, "young and middle-aged people may be able to reduce risk of diseases of aging — including senility — simply by adding high-ORAC foods to their diets."

By studying blood samples from different groups of people, the researchers concluded that you can raise the levels of antioxidants in your blood by eating more fruits and vegetables. For now, they're recommending you eat enough fruits and vegetables to total between 3,000 and 5,000 ORAC units of antioxidants daily. Since most of the foods tested scored in the hundreds, you'd have to eat many servings to reach 3,000.

But chew on this — eating just seven dried plums a day can put you well over the 3,000 mark. All the other fruits and vegetables you eat would be gravy. Just make sure you eat a variety because each fruit and vegetable has different protective nutrients.

Dried fruit caution

Dried fruits make great snacks, but they tend to have more sugar than their fresh counterparts. Take this into account if you have diabetes or are watching your weight. Otherwise, dried and fresh fruits are basically the same when it comes to nutrition.

Good sources of heart-healthy fiber

Here is a helpful chart of good sources of fiber. If you're new to fiber, pick the low-fiber choices first. Then gradually work your way up to higher amounts.

Food	Serving size	Grams of fiber
Cereals		
All Bran	1/2 cup	9
raisin bran	1 cup	7
wheat germ	1 tbsp	1
instant oatmeal	1 packet	3
Bread, pasta, grains		
oat bran muffins	1 regular muffin	3
whole wheat bread	1 slice	2
rice, brown	1 cup cooked	4
spaghetti, whole wheat	1 cup cooked	6
Fruits		
apple, with skin	1 medium	3
banana	1 medium	3
blackberries	1 cup	8
blueberries	1 cup	4
orange	1	3
dried plums	5	3
Vegetables, beans, and peas cooked		
broccoli	1 cup	5
brussels sprouts	1 cup	4
carrots	1 cup	5
sweet potato	1 medium	5
baked beans	1 cup	10
lentils	1 cup	16

4 great reasons to eat whole grains

One of the best and easiest ways to improve your health is to eat more fiber. Just trading in your bacon and egg breakfast for a bowl of cereal every morning could save your life someday.

You're not the only one who has a tough time getting enough fiber into your diet. Although recommended amounts of fiber range from 21 to 38 grams per day, most Americans only get between 5 and 20 grams daily. You can easily add more by switching from refined to whole-grain foods.

The refining process strips grains of their nutrient-rich outer layers. But whole grains are processed less so they keep their outer layers and most of their nutrition and fiber. The health benefits are real, not hype. Here's a look at what whole grains can do for you.

Cap cholesterol. Eating cereal for breakfast seems to lower blood cholesterol and cut down the amount of fat and cholesterol you eat throughout the day. Whole-grain cereals, in particular, slash LDL and total cholesterol and boost insulin control, benefits refined grains don't boast.

Snuff out heart disease. A Harvard Medical School study of 75,521 nurses showed that eating about 2.5 servings of whole grains a day could lower your risk of heart disease by about 30 percent, an estimate the researchers said may be "conservative."

Study after study reports the more whole grains you eat, the lower your risk of developing heart disease. Louis Sullivan, M.D., former Secretary of the U.S. Department of Health and Human Services, takes the research seriously. "Increasing whole grain consumption could have a profound impact on the health of the nation," he says. "We could reduce the incidences of heart disease and cancer substantially."

Of course, whole-grain foods have several heart-healthy things going for them, including fiber, folate, vitamin E, and potassium. But the beauty of eating whole foods is you don't have to figure out how each nutrient helps you — you get the combined benefits of them all.

Sidestep stroke. More women die from strokes than men. And many stroke survivors end up with permanent disability. Don't let this happen to you. Try some tabbouleh or a side of bulgur pilaf instead of potatoes, and you'll add more than just variety to your diet. Recent research says eating whole grains, like bulgur, can reduce your risk of stroke.

Researchers at Brigham and Women's Hospital in Boston analyzed information on more than 75,000 women participating in the Nurses' Health Study. They found those who ate the highest amount of whole grains cut their risk of an ischemic stroke — the kind caused by a blood clot to your brain — almost in half. Eat just a little more than one serving of whole grains every day, and you could reduce your risk of having a stroke by 30 to 40 percent. If you've never been a smoker, your risk is even lower.

Replacing refined grains, like white rice and bread, cakes, biscuits, or pizza made from white flour, with whole grains, like oatmeal, brown rice, bran, dark bread, and bulgur, can mean a longer, healthier life.

Defend against diabetes. Whole grains rich in fiber and magnesium mean added protection against adult-onset (type 2) diabetes, especially for older women.

Processing, or refining, makes the carbohydrates in grain easier to digest, so their sugar enters your bloodstream in a burst. This causes post-meal spikes in your blood sugar and insulin that, over time, can lead to type 2 diabetes.

Whole grains digest more slowly, and research shows their insoluble fiber improves insulin sensitivity and could help stave off diabetes. Eating just three servings of whole grains a day can trim your type 2 risk 20 to 30 percent. It also slashes your risk of metabolic syndrome, a group of health problems that increase your risk of diabetes, heart attack, and stroke.

Eating fiber doesn't have to be boring. The sheer variety of whole grains can spice things up — from hearty whole oats, old-fashioned oatmeal, nutty-flavored brown rice, natural popcorn, and sweet whole-grain corn. Some people even say whole-grain breads and cereals have a richer taste, too. Need more ideas? Try these on for size.

▶ Millet is high in fiber, protein, and magnesium. Look for it in cereals, or try steamed whole millet. Pet birds love it and you might, too.

▶ Barley is nearly bursting with fiber. Even the partially refined pearl barely has 5 grams of fiber per cup. Potassium-rich barley makes a satisfying breakfast cereal. It's great for soups, too.

▶ Buckwheat, bulgur, triticale, spelt, teff, and kamut are grains that can add interest to your meals. They may sound strange, but they're well worth getting to know.

Beware of whole-grain imposters

Check the ingredients list of "whole-grain" breads to make sure they're truly whole grain. If the first ingredient is "enriched wheat flour," it's not a whole-grain loaf. Bypass this pretender and move on to the next label. Look for the word "whole" in the first ingredient. Good examples include whole wheat, whole rye, whole oats, or whole barley. Oatmeal and brown rice count as whole grains, too. When you find names like these, you'll know you're getting the full fiber and nutrient benefits of whole-grain bread.

A better way to cut cholesterol

Good, old-fashioned oatmeal does more than stick to your ribs. It can help lower your cholesterol, improve blood sugar control, and even ward off colon cancer. That's because oat bran, the outer husk of the oat grain, contains tons of beta glucan. This sticky soluble fiber works by slowing down your food as it passes through your stomach and small intestine, explains Dr. Barbara Schneeman, a researcher at the USDA Agricultural Research Service and a professor at the University of California, Davis.

Beat high cholesterol. According to Schneeman, beta glucan sparks a process called "reverse cholesterol transport." By slowing down the passage of food through your intestines, this special fiber gives HDL particles more time to pick up cholesterol and carry it away to your liver for disposal.

▸ A recent Canadian study of overweight women showed that eating two oat bran muffins a day for four weeks lowered their total cholesterol.

▸ In a German study, over 200 men participated in a low-fat diet and exercise program, but some also ate oat bran. After just four weeks, the oat bran eaters not only reduced total cholesterol as much as 26 percent, they also cut LDL cholesterol by up to 30 percent. To get these results, the men ate 35 to 50 grams of oat bran daily (about six to eight tablespoons) hidden in breads, sauces, and desserts.

▸ Two more studies determined that adding two servings of oats every day, either in the form of oatmeal or oat bran cereal, can reduce your cholesterol.

However, not everyone will see the same benefit. If you have high cholesterol, you'll see a more dramatic dip than if your cholesterol levels are normal or low. Still, since even a modest reduction in cholesterol leads to a lower risk of heart disease, this is big news.

The FDA recommends getting four servings of foods containing beta glucan each day to reduce the risk of cardiovascular disease. One serving of beta glucan equals 0.75 grams, so four servings would give you 3 grams of beta glucan. Foods meeting that requirement can display this heart-healthy claim.

Adding just one serving of oats to your diet should help if you have high cholesterol. Otherwise, the amount you need depends on the form of oats you choose. For example, you have to eat three packets of instant oatmeal to get 3 grams of beta-glucan, but you only need one large bowl of oat bran cereal. Check food labels for "soluble fiber," and choose oat products with the most.

Drop-kick blood pressure. A muffin made with healthy whole grains, like oats, can drop high blood pressure like a rock. Researchers at the University of Minnesota found that eating fiber-rich, whole-grain oat cereal significantly lowered blood pressure. In fact, 73 percent of the people in the study were able to cut back on their blood pressure medication. The soluble fiber in oats did the trick. People in the study ate about three-fourths of a cup of Quaker Oatmeal and a cup and a third of Quaker Oat Squares each day.

Rein in diabetes. If you're struggling with diabetes, you know you should watch your carbohydrates. One good way to do that is to eat more soluble fiber. Because it's sticky and slow-moving, beta glucan slows the absorption of carbohydrates in your digestive tract. This means your blood doesn't get flooded with glucose all at once, so you don't have an immediate and urgent demand for insulin. The result – fewer spikes in blood sugar and insulin.

Many experts recommend a high-fiber diet, with an emphasis on soluble and cereal fibers, as an effective way to control diabetes. A study in *The New England Journal of Medicine* found that a diet with 50 grams of daily fiber (25 grams each of soluble and insoluble) helped keep blood sugar, insulin, and cholesterol under control in people with type 2 diabetes. It also showed you could achieve this type of diet without taking fiber supplements or eating special fiber-fortified foods.

Cut colon cancer risk. Oat bran may protect against colon cancer as well. Once again, beta-glucan does the dirty work by speeding waste products through the large intestine before they have time to do damage. Beta-glucan may also react with tiny organisms to form compounds that protect the colon wall and tame substances that can cause cancer.

Amazingly easy ways to get more fiber

It's easy to find room for more fiber in your diet. Just replace some of your favorite low-fiber foods with high-fiber substitutes like these.

Instead of:	Eat:
orange juice	whole orange
cornflakes	raisin bran
white bread	bran muffin
white rice	brown rice
meat	beans
potato chips, other snacks	carrots, celery sticks
regular cookies	whole-grain cookies

Healthy breakfast fights heart disease

Do you want an easy way to follow the American Heart Association's recommendations for a heart-healthy diet? Just eat two bowls of high-fiber cereal every day.

In a recent study, men who ate two servings of high-fiber cereal each day – one for breakfast and one later in the day as a snack – changed their diets enough to meet the AHA's recommendations for fat and cholesterol. Eating cereal for breakfast meant they ate fewer fatty breakfast foods, like omelets, pastries, and breakfast sandwiches. And some of the men ate cereal as an after-dinner snack, instead of their usual bowl of ice cream.

Researchers didn't tell them to make any changes except adding the cereal to their regular diets, but the men found that they automatically ate fewer fatty foods because the fiber was so filling. Two more studies showed similar results.

▶ In a six-year Harvard study of fiber intake involving more than 40,000 men, those who ate the most cereal fiber drastically lowered their risk of heart disease. The more they ate, the more their cholesterol came down. For every additional 10 grams (g) of cereal fiber the men ate, their risk of heart disease dropped an astounding 29 percent.

▶ One study showed that men who ate 29 g of fiber a day, roughly the amount in three cups of Grape Nuts cereal, were 43 percent less likely to have a stroke as those who ate only about half that much. Cereal fiber, the kind in oats, wheat, rye, and barley, gave the most protection.

What's more, cereal fiber is especially good at warding off diabetes. Fiber, in general, helps prevent diabetes because it slows down the conversion of carbohydrates into glucose, says Diana H. Noren, R.D., a certified diabetes counselor in Georgia. Also, if you eat a high-fiber carbohydrate, your body will respond with less insulin than it would if you eat a low-fiber food, she says. This is better for your overall health because high insulin levels could lead to weight gain and high blood pressure, among other problems.

In a study of nearly 36,000 older women in Iowa, the ones who ate several daily servings of high-fiber foods had a significantly lower risk of developing diabetes than women who ate little fiber.

The women in the study who ate more than 7.5 g of cereal fiber per day were 36 percent less likely to get diabetes than women who ate less than half that amount. And 7.5 g is not a lot of fiber. A 1-ounce serving of bran flakes for breakfast will supply you with more than 8 g of cereal fiber. Noren says you can actually eat a little more of a cereal that's high in fiber without harming your total carbohydrate count.

Sweep out cholesterol with wheat germ

The word "germ" probably makes you think of sickness and disease. But put the word "wheat" in front of it, and you have a whole new ballgame.

Wheat germ is made from cut-up flakes of wheat berry, the heart of the wheat kernel, and it's jam-packed with protein, fiber, polyunsaturated fat, vitamins, and minerals. It's the most nutritionally dense part of the wheat kernel, which also includes the endosperm and bran, or outer husk.

Chances are you get plenty of wheat in your diet since most breads are made with that grain. But you probably don't eat much wheat germ, one of the healthiest parts of the kernel, because it is often removed during milling. That's too bad, because wheat germ can lower cholesterol and help your heart.

Cholesterol has the power to clog or block your arteries, trigger heart attacks, and cause stroke. But wheat germ has the raw power to stop it. You can dissolve cholesterol and open up arteries with just a quarter of a cup of wheat germ daily.

A French study found that eating 30 grams, or about a quarter of a cup, of raw wheat germ a day for 14 weeks lowered total cholesterol by 7.2 percent. It also lowered LDL or "bad" cholesterol by 15.4 percent and triglycerides, another type of blood fat, by 11.3 percent. This is important because, according to another study, reducing cholesterol just 7 percent may slice your risk of heart disease 15 percent.

Wheat germ's success against LDL cholesterol could stem from the antioxidant powers of vitamin E. Dr. Lori J. Mosca of the University of Michigan led a study that suggested vitamin E from foods, but not from supplements, prevented LDL particles from becoming oxidized and forming plaque in your blood vessels.

Vitamin E in supplements typically doesn't have the same balance of mixed tocopherols — alpha, beta, gamma, and delta — found naturally in foods. What's more, taking large amounts of vitamin E supplements can excessively thin the blood and apparently caused higher death rates in a recent study.

Your best bet is to get vitamin E through your diet. "We can never be sure exactly which nutrient is providing the benefits, and it is likely that several different nutrients are involved," Mosca explains. "That's why we recommend getting vitamin E from foods."

Wheat germ contains all four types of tocopherols. You can find it in both toasted and natural forms. Mix a little wheat germ into your next bowl of cereal or yogurt. Its nutty flavor makes a great addition to cereals, pancake and waffle mixes, biscuit and bread recipes, and meatloaf.

Look for wheat germ in jars in health food and grocery stores. Keep it in a handy place in the fridge for a quick sprinkle on your favorite foods. Use it soon after you buy it because its oiliness makes it turn rancid quickly. You can also buy wheat germ oil, but it has a strong flavor and is fairly expensive.

What 'organic' really means

Organic food contains fewer pesticide residues than conventional food, but you pay extra for that benefit. If you choose to shop for organic foods, learn how to read the labels. Use these guidelines to see just how organic a product is, so you'll always know exactly what you're paying for.

- ▶ 100 percent organic — no synthetic pesticides, herbicides, chemical fertilizers, antibiotics, hormones, additives, or preservatives

- ▶ organic — contains 95 percent or more organically produced ingredients

- ▶ made with organic ingredients — at least 70 percent of the product is organic

If less than 70 percent of the product is organic, the word "organic" can't appear on the front of the package, but it can appear in the list of ingredients. Look for the USDA organic label on a product to feel confident you're getting the most natural product possible.

An apple a day keeps heart disease at bay

Students who bring their teacher an apple are doing more than seeking favor – they're giving the teacher an "A" in heart health. Apples are great foods for all-around heart health. Not only are they high in fiber, vitamins, minerals, and antioxidants, they're also fat-free, cholesterol-free, and low in sodium. The magnesium and potassium in apples help regulate your blood pressure and keep your heart beating steadily.

Apples also contain the flavonoid quercetin, a naturally occurring antioxidant that protects your artery walls from damage and keeps your blood flowing smoothly. In fact, adding flavonoid-rich foods, like apples, to your diet has been scientifically confirmed to lower your risk of heart disease. So an apple a day really might keep the doctor away.

Clobbers high cholesterol. Apples are packed with pectin, a natural form of soluble fiber that can lower your cholesterol up to 30 percent if you eat it every day. The soluble fiber in this sweet, crunchy fruit grabs on to LDL cholesterol and hustles it out of your body before it gets absorbed in your gut and ends up clogging your arteries. If you want to lower your cholesterol with soluble fiber, experts say you should get results by eating 6 to 40 grams of pectin every day. One delicious apple provides 1.5 grams.

Cuts your risk of heart disease. Sometimes it's hard to remember which food is good for which part of your body. The next time you pick up an apple, examine it carefully. It's shaped a bit like a heart – and that should help you remember apples are good for your heart.

It's the magnesium and potassium in apples that help regulate your blood pressure and keep your heart beating steadily, and it's the flavonoid quercetin, a naturally occurring antioxidant, that protects your artery walls from damage and keeps your blood flowing smoothly.

In fact, adding flavonoid-rich foods, like apples, to your diet has been scientifically proven to lower your risk of heart disease. There's proof of this in a study of Japanese women who ate foods high in quercetin. They were less likely to get heart disease than other women, and they had lower levels of total and LDL, or bad, cholesterol.

Strikes at the heart of strokes. Apples are even a smart choice for helping avoid strokes. Scientists aren't sure which ingredient in this multi-talented fruit to credit, but the connection is clear – people who regularly eat apples are less likely to have strokes than people who don't.

Keeps your body young. Antioxidants can protect you from many of the diseases that seem to be a part of aging. In fact, so many people are taking supplements for antioxidant protection that it's become a multibillion-dollar industry. But the evidence is mounting that whole foods can do more for you than pills.

When scientists compared a 1,500-milligram vitamin C supplement to one small apple, the results were astounding – the antioxidant values were equal. That means a fresh apple has more than 15 times the antioxidant power of the recommended daily amount of vitamin C. Why waste money on flavorless supplements when you can get better antioxidant firepower from munching on a crunchy fruit?

Chop bad cholesterol with marinades

Marinating your meat will help keep it from forming unhealthy cholesterol oxidation products during cooking, which can lead to heart disease and cancer. According to one study, an effective marinade mixes 10 percent soy sauce, 1 percent sugar, and 89 percent water. You can convert that to 10 tablespoons (5 ounces) soy sauce, 1 tablespoon sugar, and 5 1/2 cups of water.

Pick the best proteins

Protein is a part of every cell in your body, and no other nutrient plays as many different roles in keeping you alive and healthy. It is important for the growth and repair of your muscles, bones, skin, tendons, ligaments, hair, eyes, and other tissues. Without it, you would lack the enzymes and hormones you need for metabolism, digestion, and other important processes.

Your body needs many different proteins for various purposes. It makes them from about 20 "building blocks" called amino acids. Nine of these are essential amino acids, which means you must get them from food. The others are nonessential. This doesn't mean you don't need them. You just don't have to eat them because your body can make them.

Heart-smart protein

High-protein sources, like meat, are often high in fat, too. If you don't watch the fat content, you risk weight gain, heart disease, and worsening diabetes. Get heart-smart protein with these lean choices.

▸ Focus on fish, skinless turkey, and chicken. They're lower in fat than beef and pork. Legumes and tofu (soybean curd) offer other low-fat protein choices.

▸ Choose beef cuts with "loin" or "round" in the name.

▸ Pick "choice" instead of "prime," and choose cuts graded "USDA Select."

▸ When buying pork, pick cuts with the word "loin" or "leg" in the name.

▸ Give up frying your food. Bake, broil, roast, or microwave it instead.

▸ Eat only low-fat or fat-free dairy products. You'll get the same nutrients, including dairy protein, without the saturated fat.

Meat, poultry, fish, and dairy foods pack the most protein. Animal protein is also complete, meaning it contains all the essential amino acids. Next, come legumes — beans, peas, and peanuts. Their protein is incomplete, because they lack some essential amino acids. Soybeans are the exception, since they provide all the essential amino acids.

Protein is so important to your body's survival, you may think you need to eat a lot of it. Not true. Moderate amounts of protein may help balance your blood sugar. Unlike most refined carbohydrates, protein does not cause glucose levels to spike, making it a smart choice at mealtime.

Unfortunately, most Americans already get twice as much protein as they need — mostly from meat. The typical Western diet includes about 100 grams of protein, while 50 grams is closer to what your body needs. All the excess can put a strain on your kidneys and liver and make it more difficult for your body to absorb other nutrients. Not to mention, eating lots of meat can also mean eating lots of saturated fat and cholesterol — two things your heart definitely doesn't need.

Start paying attention to how much protein you eat by reading the nutrition label on foods when possible. And make a conscious effort to get more of your protein from legumes and grains if you usually eat lots of meat, especially red meat. You'll learn more about the most heart friendly protein sources in the next few pages. Until then, these tips can help you make the most of this important nutrient.

▶ Get complete protein from plants by eating any two or more of these plant foods, with or without beans — grains, seeds and nuts, and vegetables. You don't have to eat them in the same dish, or even in the same meal. But many cultures have created combinations that work well, like corn and beans in Mexico, or rice and split peas in India, or peanut butter sandwiches in America.

▶ Cooking with moist rather than dry heat, perhaps boiled in a stew rather than fried, or soaking meat in a marinade using wine, lemon juice, or vinegar makes the protein easier to digest.

▶ Plan more of your meals around fruits, vegetables, and grains. For example, dishes that combine beans and rice are filling and high in protein. Also, consider replacing some of the meat protein in your diet with soy-based foods, like tofu.

▶ You don't have to cut out meat altogether – just choose lean cuts and eat smaller portions. Fish and skinless turkey and chicken are lower in fat than beef and pork. And don't stop eating calcium-rich dairy products. Simply pick low-fat or fat-free varieties.

'Cheap' way to clobber cholesterol

"Beans, beans, good for your heart. If you eat them, it shows you're smart." OK, so that's not the way the rhyme goes, but it's true. You'd be hard pressed to find a more cost-effective, nutrient-packed vegetable than beans.

"Beans are an excellent source of protein, vitamins, and minerals," says Dr. James Anderson, a medical professor at the University of Kentucky and author of the *High-Fiber Fitness Plan.* "Beans are naturally low in fat and provide more protein per penny than any other food. They are also great sources of both soluble and insoluble fiber," which helps you stay regular and keeps a lid on both cholesterol and blood sugar. They even have lots of phytochemicals – antioxidants that can help prevent cancer.

Filled with fiber. It just goes to show you, some of the healthiest foods are actually the cheapest. This 50¢ meal can help you lose weight and lower your cholesterol without even trying. That's what 24 men did. As part of a university study, these men ate about 2 1/2 cups of canned beans, a good source of fiber, each day for three weeks. They lost weight and lowered their cholesterol without cutting calories or otherwise changing their diets.

Anderson says the soluble fiber in beans removes extra cholesterol from your body, and it keeps your body from producing too much cholesterol. Plus, beans fill you up without lots of calories – only

225 calories in a one-cup serving. Your body also takes a long time to absorb these high-fiber foods, so you feel fuller longer.

Packed with protein. By providing plenty of protein without artery-clogging cholesterol and saturated fat, beans and other legumes make wonderful alternatives to meat. If you switch just half of your protein intake from meat to legume sources, you could lower your cholesterol by 10 percent or more. And when your protein comes from beans and other vegetables instead of always from meat, you improve your chances of avoiding cancer and liver damage.

Bursting with antioxidants. You've probably heard about all the high-powered antioxidants in fruits like blueberries and blackberries – and how they may help protect you from such dangers as heart disease, cancer, and perhaps even aging. But a fascinating new study suggests black beans may have a pretty hefty antioxidant stockpile of their own.

What's more, these antioxidants include health-building plant pigments, like anthocyanins, the same family of heavy-hitter nutrients found in blueberries and blackberries. Stay tuned to find out what exciting new health benefits these black bean antioxidants may hold in store for you.

If you are fairly new to bean eating, here are some delicious ways to easily add beans to your meals.

▶ Start with canned beans. They come in many varieties and flavors and require little effort to prepare. "Canned beans cook more quickly and are also a nutritious alternative to dried beans," says Anderson. "They can be easily added to many soups, stews, and casseroles."

▶ You can easily add beans to your diet by tossing them into every soup recipe, mixing them into your salads, and topping potatoes with chili instead of butter and cheese.

▶ To save time later, take a little extra time once a week and cook up a pot of dried beans. That way, they'll be ready and waiting for you to add to a soup or serve cold on a salad.

▶ Nutritionists are trying to get the word out that you can eat beans and have friends, too. You can easily reduce the amount of gas legumes produce by changing the water a few times while you're boiling them. Another alternative is to add a product called Beano to legumes after cooking. A few drops are all it takes to make them "wind free."

Leaner, meaner ground meat

After cooking ground meat, blot it with paper towels, then put it in a colander and rinse with hot water. You've just "bathed" out about half the fat. Or microwave your hamburger patties for one to three minutes, then pour off the liquid and grill as usual. Choose reduced-fat or fat-free cheeses to top that hamburger, and pair it with oven-roasted potatoes instead of french fries. For other types of red meat, choose lean cuts, trim off any excess fat, and use low-fat cooking methods, like broiling, roasting, or grilling. Your heart will heave a sigh of relief.

Enjoy the health benefits of the Asian diet

Eastern cultures have long boasted some of the best overall health records in the world. For centuries, the people of Japan, China, Thailand, and Vietnam have enjoyed delicious, exotic meals, while managing to avoid many of the pitfalls of the Western diet.

The low-fat, high-fiber makeup of these diets, combined with more active, physically demanding lifestyles, offer a much better defense against heart disease. People from Asian nations also enjoy lower rates of many types of cancer. But how can you enjoy the health benefits of the Asian diet without moving to China? The answer is as simple as one little bean.

The soybean is actually a legume, like a pea or lentil, and is a common staple of almost all Asian diets. Like other beans, it's rich in essential B vitamins, and it's an excellent source of both soluble and insoluble fiber. Plus, it's loaded with artery-loving omega-3 fats and provides all of the essential proteins. And soy protein packs more vitamins and minerals than either meat or dairy proteins.

Past studies suggested the protein in soy helped lower cholesterol, especially when combined with a low-fat diet. A review by the American Heart Association of 22 soy studies didn't find a link between soy protein and cholesterol. However, the researchers say soy foods could still help your heart if you eat them in place of red meat and high-fat dairy products. That's because soy protein has no saturated fat and more heart-healthy polyunsaturated fats and nutrients than either meat or dairy products.

Here's something else to keep in mind – researchers in Hawaii concluded that soy may contribute to brain aging after examining the diets of more than 8,000 Japanese-American men for over 30 years. They found that those who ate two or more servings of tofu, or soybean curd, a week were much more likely to become forgetful as they grew older compared with men who ate little or no tofu.

The more tofu the subjects ate, the more learning and memory problems they suffered in later life. Loss of mental function occurred in 4 percent of the men who ate the least amount of tofu compared with 19 percent of the men who ate the greatest amount of tofu. In view of that study, any consumption of soy should be in great moderation.

Experts don't recommend taking soy isoflavone supplements – antioxidant compounds isolated from soy foods that are implicated in memory loss – since they seem to have no impact on cholesterol.

Try using soy flour or soy milk in your baking, or add a little tofu to your salad. But don't just add soy products to a typical American diet. Most Americans eat too much protein already, and if you add protein-rich soybeans to a meat-heavy diet, you're likely to have kidney trouble. Your kidneys will have to work overtime to excrete all the waste produced when your body metabolizes protein.

Soy flour baking tip

You can substitute one cup of soy flour plus one-fourth cup potato starch in place of one cup wheat flour in recipes.

Antioxidants — secret weapons stop cell damage

You've heard antioxidants are good for you, but you may be surprised to learn just how much you need them. When your body processes the oxygen you breathe, it produces unstable compounds called free radicals at the same time.

These compounds are unstable because they lack an electron, a tiny atomic particle. In an effort to balance themselves, free radicals travel through your body like a band of pickpockets, trying to steal electrons from stable, healthy cells. When they succeed, they leave the cell irreversibly damaged.

One damaged cell is no big deal. But over time, lots of these pickpocket molecules can cause so much damage, called oxidation, that your body becomes weak. In fact, researchers have linked free radical damage to over 200 diseases, including cataracts, diabetes, heart disease, and some cancers.

Luckily, you can stop the damage with nutritional allies known as antioxidants. They fight oxidation by combining with free radicals or giving them an electron, making them stable. Your body produces some antioxidants itself, but you can also get loads of them from fresh fruits and vegetables.

That's one reason the American Heart Association recommends eating at least five servings of fruits and vegetables every day. Fresh fruits and vegetables are loaded with antioxidants, which may prevent LDL cholesterol from becoming oxidized. That's important because, once oxidized, LDL cholesterol makes a beeline for your artery walls much faster.

Dr. Lori J. Mosca, director of preventive cardiology research and education at the University of Michigan, says, "When a fat such as LDL undergoes oxidation, it is more prone to collect in blood vessels to form plaque. Over time, the plaque narrows the blood vessels, or unleashes a blood clot, which can result in a heart attack or stroke." In fact, some scientists believe LDL cholesterol only harms you once it becomes oxidized. "When LDL is not oxidized, it does not seem to cause problems."

Tart berry guards your arteries

Drinking red wine or grape juice can be good for your heart, but drinking cranberry juice might be even better. The antioxidants, flavonoids, and polyphenols in cranberries can help protect you from heart disease.

University researchers' shocking findings are great news for Americans. This amazing berry opened up hardened arteries in recent studies by relaxing blood vessels and preventing LDL cholesterol from forming plaques.

Researchers at the University of Wisconsin gave cranberry juice powder to animals with atherosclerosis for six months, and it helped blood flow by relaxing their blood vessels. Dr. Ted Wilson, a professor at the University of Wisconsin–La Crosse, discovered cranberry juice also prevents low-density lipoprotein (LDL) cholesterol, or "bad" cholesterol, from becoming oxidized.

That's big news in the heart world. "What LDL cholesterol does is deliver cholesterol into the arterial wall," Wilson says. "And when LDL gets oxidized, LDL is delivered to the arterial wall much, much, much more rapidly. Once it's oxidized, it gets taken up and forms a plaque. And those plaques are what obstructs blood flow to your heart and your brain." When you stop LDL oxidation, you slow down the process. That gives the LDL cholesterol less of a chance to stick to your arteries and clog them.

"The particular flavonoids in cranberry juice are particularly good at providing antioxidants and opening up or dilating blood vessels," Wilson says. He also speculates that, because of this, cranberry juice might be able to prevent blood clotting.

But flavonoids are only the beginning. Cranberries are also high in fiber, which lowers cholesterol and helps reduce your risk of heart disease and stroke. And don't forget about potassium, which keeps your blood pressure under control, and vitamin C, the powerful antioxidant that fights atherosclerosis, high blood pressure, and stroke.

So how effective is cranberry juice when it comes to protecting your heart? "In comparison to red wine or grape juice, very comparable or better," Wilson says. And here's the best part – one glass a day might do the trick. These tart, high-fiber treats are very high in antioxidants, according to a study by University of Scranton professor Joe Vinson. "Cranberries are one of the healthiest fruits. I think people should eat more of them," Vinson says.

Get the benefits and tart taste by sprinkling dried cranberries over a bowl of oatmeal, barley, or other cereal. If you like your cranberry in a glass, look for products with the highest percentage of cranberry juice and the least sugar or corn syrup.

Green tea's cousin cleans arteries, too

Would you believe four weeks to cleaner arteries — just by drinking a few cups of black tea daily? If you have heart disease, you know you run a greater risk of having a stroke. But adding a simple and relaxing habit might change the numbers in your favor. While most people may have heard that green tea has lots of health benefits, black tea is no slacker. Research shows that drinking black tea can help open up narrow blood vessels.

When volunteers drank four cups of tea daily for four weeks, their blood vessels expanded to near normal size. The changes took place within just a few hours of drinking the first cup of tea. Another study found drinking three cups of black tea for four weeks helped arteries resist the build up of cholesterol.

Powerful brew renews blood vessels

It's hard to believe something as soothing as a warm cup of tea could protect you from heart disease, heart attacks, and stroke, but it's true. A health secret among the Asian world for thousands of years, now you can learn how to make green tea work for you.

According to legend, the Chinese Emperor Shen-Nung discovered this tasty drink by accident in 2737 B.C. As the story goes, the emperor was boiling a kettle of water on a terrace when some leaves from a nearby bush happened to drift by and fall into the water.

The emperor tasted the brew and found it delicious. It wasn't long before people were adding the leaves to kettles all over the Far East and enjoying the protective benefits of this plant.

Both black and green teas are made from the same bush, *Camellia sinensis*, native to China and India. Green tea is different only in how it's processed. Unlike black tea, which is fermented, green tea leaves are steamed soon after being picked. This steaming process helps preserve the plant's antioxidants.

Many scientists believe green tea antioxidants are more powerful than those found in most vegetables. Green tea also contains B vitamins and vitamin C and is lower in caffeine than black tea. Because of the powerful ability of its antioxidants to fight cell-damaging free radicals, this simple drink can help renew your veins and arteries naturally.

Heads off heart attacks. You may want to think twice about your next cup of coffee and brew some green tea instead. A Harvard Medical School study found that tea drinkers had a lower risk of heart attack than java lovers. Meanwhile, a Japanese study showed that people who drank at least one cup of green tea a day were 42 percent less likely to have a heart attack than those who didn't. Scientists think theanine – an amino acid in green tea – makes blood less sticky so it can move smoothly through your arteries.

Clamps down on cholesterol. High cholesterol increases your risk of heart disease, but regular tea consumption may help keep cholesterol under control. One Japanese study that followed tea drinkers over the course of nearly five years showed that having several cups of green tea a day reduced cholesterol and triglyceride levels significantly.

Lowers high blood pressure. You can drop your blood pressure naturally if you start by drinking this delicious tea. Researchers in Taiwan studied the effects of green tea in more than 1,500 people. They concluded that drinking a half-cup (4 ounces) to two-and-a-half-cups (20 ounces) of moderate-strength green tea every day for a year reduced the participants' risk of developing high blood pressure by 46 percent.

Beats heart disease. Another study in the Netherlands found that older men who consumed the most fruits, vegetables, and tea were the least likely to die from heart disease or stroke. Loaded with flavonoids, especially compounds called catechins, tea dilates arteries, easing the inflammation associated with atherosclerosis, thereby improving blood flow. Antioxidants also fight harmful free radicals, the molecules scientists suspect contribute to heart disease. Other researchers believe green tea's protective effect may come from its ability to lower blood pressure or LDL cholesterol, both risk factors for heart disease. Whatever the reason, it seems to work.

Stops stroke damage. An ordinary chemical in green tea, called gallotannin, might wind up becoming an extraordinary means of avoiding brain damage after a stroke. Normally, brain cells die from destructive free radicals unleashed during a stroke. But gallotannin blocks a certain chemical chain reaction and, as a result, keeps these critical cells alive. To get the greatest effect, drink two to five cups a day.

Serve the perfect cup of green tea

Follow these brewing tips to make the most of this healthy beverage. Use 8 ounces of fresh, good-quality water for every heaping teaspoon of green tea. Steep it in water that is hot, but not boiling, for two to three minutes. Boiling water destroys some of the antioxidants in tea. Plus, you'll end up with bitter tea if you steep it too long or if the water is too hot. Store tea leaves in a dark, airtight container, and keep the container in a cool, dry place. Use the leaves within a month or two to get the best health benefits.

Juicy fruit fends off illness

Oddly enough, the orange didn't get its name from its color but rather from an ancient Sanskrit word meaning "fragrant." In fact, people have prized this golden fruit for its beauty and scent for thousands of years.

Originally from Southeast Asia, oranges made their way to warm-weather areas of Europe, North Africa, and the United States. In 1513, Ponce de Leon planted the first orange tree in Florida, an area that now produces most of the world's oranges.

In the 1700s, oranges became even more popular when a Scottish naval surgeon discovered oranges and other citrus fruits cured scurvy, the plague of seamen everywhere.

Of course, oranges do much more than ward off a nutritional deficiency. Studies show orange juice can lower blood pressure, help fight cancer, and boost your brainpower, thanks to its vast stores of vitamin C, carotenoids, folate, fiber, and potassium. And don't forget how sweet, juicy, and delicious oranges are. Peel one and sink your teeth in. Now "orange" you glad you did?

Guards your heart. Just as a single orange has several juicy sections, all oranges have many powerful weapons to fight heart disease. In fact, eating just one extra serving a day of mouth-watering citrus fruit can reduce strokes, lower obesity, and fight heart disease. Studies have shown a daily serving of citrus fruits, like oranges, can bring down your risk of stroke by nearly 20 percent.

▶ Fiber, especially the soluble kind in fruit, helps lower cholesterol. Too much cholesterol can clog or block your arteries, leading to atherosclerosis, heart attack, or stroke. You get 3 grams of fiber per orange.

▶ Folate neutralizes homocysteine, a dangerous substance that increases clotting and can damage the lining of your blood vessels. One small orange provides around 30 micrograms (mcg) of folate.

▶ Potassium helps keep your blood pressure under control – especially when you limit your sodium intake – and lowers your risk for stroke. An orange has about 237 mg of potassium and no sodium.

▶ Vitamin C may lower your blood pressure, improve blood flow, and shrink your risk of stroke. Because it's an antioxidant, it may fight cholesterol by preventing bad LDL cholesterol from becoming oxidized and, consequently, more dangerous to your artery walls. Vitamin C also counteracts inflammation and boosts levels of beneficial HDL cholesterol.

As a bonus, eating fruit on a regular basis can help you avoid weight gain. A 12-year study of thousands of women revealed that the ones who ate the most fruit were less likely to become obese during middle age. Now that's a sweet deal.

Cancels out cancer. Cancer might be called "the Big C," but that title rightfully belongs to vitamin C, which looms large in the battle against the disease.

Although some tests have shown large doses (10 grams) of vitamin C can treat people with cancer and help them live longer, the antioxidant vitamin mainly shields you from free radicals that can cause cancer. Studies indicate vitamin C may protect you from stomach, throat, lung, bladder, and pancreatic cancers.

Oranges also provide fiber, folate, flavonoids, and the carotenoid beta-cryptoxanthin – all dedicated cancer enemies. With all that protection, it's easy to see why eating more of this fruit is a sensible anti-cancer strategy.

Mends your memory. Free radicals, remember, are unstable molecules your body makes as it processes oxygen. They zip around damaging your cells and making you more likely to fall prey to health problems – like memory loss. Luckily, antioxidants, substances in certain foods, get rid of free radicals.

According to scientists at the USDA-ARS Human Nutrition Research Center on Aging, your brain needs antioxidants to keep sharp. Otherwise, its cells wear down after years of free radical bombardment. Your memory becomes a little fuzzier, just like the picture in an old television.

Your best sources of antioxidants are vitamin E, vitamin C, beta carotene, and flavonoids. All together, the USDA experts believe these antioxidants can fix free radical damage done in the past, as well as prevent damage in the future. Fruits and vegetables pack an arsenal of antioxidants. So, eat strawberries, blueberries, prunes, brussels sprouts, and kale. They're like television repairmen for your head.

If, despite a healthy menu, you or someone you know experiences a serious memory loss, see a doctor. It may be a sign of a bigger problem, like Alzheimer's disease. With professional help, you can chart a course of treatment.

Orange juice – Is fresh really best?

Surprisingly, fresh oranges may not be the best way to get the most vitamin C. The amount of vitamin C in oranges differs from one variety to the next. In addition, it breaks down over time and with changing temperatures.

A recent study found frozen orange juice concentrate may be your best source. Researchers examined different brands of frozen concentrate and ready-to-drink cartons of orange juice. They found that the frozen juice mixed with water contained more vitamin C than ready-to-drink juices. Plus, it retained the vitamin longer.

Next time you visit the grocery store, head to the frozen-food aisle to pick up your OJ. You'll not only save money over ready-to-drink brands, you'll get more vitamin C for your buck.

Little fruit packs big punch

If you're looking for a quick, delicious snack, it's hard to do better than the little apricot. This single fruit can help your heart; fight fatigue; improve your skin, hair, and nails; regulate blood pressure; keep digestion moving smoothly; and even help produce estrogen. The best part? It only has about 16 calories.

Alexander the Great fell in love with this surprisingly sweet fruit in Asia, where he found them growing wild. When he returned to Europe from his military expeditions, he brought some with him.

The ancient Romans gave the apricot its name – from the Latin word for "precocious" – because the apricot is the first fruit of the season to ripen. The name stuck, and the apricot spread all over, from Europe, to America, and all the way to Australia.

No wonder. It's a fantastic fruit jam-packed with beta carotene, iron, fiber, vitamin C, boron, potassium, and several B vitamins. If you dry an apricot, its nutrients get more concentrated, making dried apricots a great snack.

Halts heart disease. Eating dried apricots as a snack can punch up your levels of iron, potassium, beta carotene, magnesium, and copper. These important nutrients help control your blood pressure and prevent heart disease. The potassium alone protects your blood vessels from damage, prevents dangerous irregular heartbeats, and keeps your blood pressure down. Plus, as few as five dried apricots can give you up to 3 grams of fiber, which sweeps cholesterol out of your system before it has a chance to clog your arteries.

Lengthens your life. Believe it or not, some people claim apricots are the secret to living to age 120. They get this idea from the Hunzas, a tribe living in the Himalayan Mountains of Asia who are somewhat long lived, but they don't have quite the longevity some have claimed. Common health problems, like cancer, heart disease, high blood pressure, and high cholesterol, appear to be less frequent in Hunza. And researchers are wondering if apricots, a main part of their diet, are partly responsible. The Hunzas eat fresh apricots in season and dry the rest to eat during their long, cold winter.

Although eating apricots can't guarantee you'll live a long life, recent research suggests the little fruit may help you live a better life.

The B vitamins in dried apricots may protect you from Alzheimer's disease and age-related mental problems, like memory loss.

The iron in apricots can help fight fatigue and hair loss, while the fiber keeps your bowels moving smoothly. The boron in apricots and prunes may naturally help your body make estrogen and absorb calcium, while its vast stores of vitamin E and beta carotene, which your body converts to vitamin A, make for healthier skin and nails.

Dried apricots beat fresh apricots hands down when it comes to a number of important nutrients. The dried variety has more than three times the amount of fiber and beta carotene. That's a lot of punch in one chewy, portable package.

But fresh, juicy apricots still provide a nutritional bang and can really hit the spot. Look for fresh apricots from California and Washington on your grocer's shelves during June, July, and August. Slice them up in fruit salads, purée them for sauces, make preserves, peel and slice them in yogurt or on ice cream, or whip up an apricot tart.

Fish and garlic make heart-smart duo

Try these two healthful tidbits that really taste great together. Fish, rich in omega-3 fatty acids, and garlic, full of sulfur compounds, team up to fight cholesterol. This dynamic food duo lowers your LDL better together than either one can do alone. A recent Indian study found that the combination of fish oil capsules and garlic supplements lowered LDL by 21 percent and boosted HDL by 5 percent. Serve up some garlicky fish for dinner. Your cholesterol will improve.

4 ways garlic keeps you healthy

Some people say a clove of garlic a day keeps health problems away. According to garlic grower Loyd Hubbard of the Gnos Garlic Company, it's true. "Garlic is a natural antibiotic and detoxifier," says Hubbard. "In addition, it can purify the blood naturally and lower blood cholesterol."

This one "miracle plant" can attack atherosclerosis, battle cholesterol, bring down blood pressure, banish bacteria, and crush blood clots. Seasoning with this delicious herb may even help you throw away your saltshaker. Garlic is the number three spice used in America, but its strengths go far beyond its use as a savory food seasoning. In fact, it may protect you from just about everything, from the common cold to heart disease.

Why is garlic so special? Crushing it produces a powerful, penicillin-like compound called allicin. The allicin breaks down to create several sulfur compounds plus a substance called ajoene, giving garlic its distinctive smell. In addition, garlic is a good source of selenium, and it's chock-full of antioxidants that protect your body. Here are four ways garlic helps wallop health problems.

Attacks atherosclerosis. The buildup of cholesterol in the heart's arteries is the leading cause of death in the Western world. Garlic helps to lower cholesterol and blood pressure, protecting the heart's arteries from potential disaster.

Controls cholesterol. Slash your cholesterol – without drugs – just by eating two vegetables you can grow right in your garden. Garlic goes after your bad LDL cholesterol without harming your good HDL cholesterol. Garlic's cousin, the onion, may also lower cholesterol. Onions have plenty of flavonoids, including quercetin, which stop LDL cholesterol from oxidizing and blocking your arteries.

Lowers blood pressure. Garlic lowers cholesterol, which allows your blood to flow more freely through your arteries. That means lower blood pressure and less stress on your heart.

Crushes clots. Ajoene, along with other compounds, makes blood less sticky and reduces the formation of harmful clots. This also allows your blood to keep flowing, reducing your risk of heart attack or stroke.

Add to this list garlic's power as a potent antibiotic that kills a variety of bacteria, fungi, mold, yeasts, and parasites. Some of garlic's victims include *H. pylori, Salmonella, Staphylococcus, E. coli,* and *Candida.* Not to mention it can boost your immune system so you're less likely to get sick with colds or flu. So don't reach for that box of tissues – grab some garlic instead.

All these benefits are a boost to your health, but if you don't like the taste, you probably won't eat it. So what's the best-tasting garlic to cook with? Hubbard recommends elephant garlic, which is considered the Vidalia onion of garlic because you can eat the bulb raw. "Elephant garlic is the best garlic to cook with," Hubbard says. "It has a smoother, milder, sweeter flavor that doesn't overpower the main dish. It's the specialty garlic for the connoisseur. Some of our best customers are executive chefs in four-star restaurants."

Thinking of buying garlic supplements? "Traditional Chinese medicine has used garlic for thousands of years," says Christopher Gardner, Ph.D., of Stanford University's Prevention Research Center. "They didn't use garlic pills. They used real garlic."

That may be your best bet, too. Recently, a consumer organization tested the quality of supplements. They found that the amount of allicin you get from the recommended daily serving of each brand varied wildly.

The clinical trials that tested fresh garlic for atherosclerosis or high cholesterol used 2 to 4 grams of fresh garlic a day – about one clove. Add it to an Asian vegetable stir-fry, a Mediterranean salad, or another heart-healthy dish. When cooking with fresh garlic, mince or crush it first, then wait 10 to 15 minutes before cooking it to get the full health benefits. Avoid cooking it at high heats, since that can destroy its heart-healthy compounds.

If you take medication, talk with your doctor before ramping up your garlic intake since this herb enhances the effects of some drugs, like blood thinners.

Delicious drink fends off heart disease

Taking aspirin for your arteries? A delicious daily glass of grape juice may work just as well. After years of taking grapes apart and examining the pieces, scientists have decided they are healthiest just as they are — whole.

Grape seed extract and grape skin extract each, on its own, does little to stop your blood from clotting and blocking your arteries. But when the two substances are combined, the mixture can reduce platelet clumping by 91 percent. And that's why grape juice, made from whole grapes, is a heart-smart choice. Studies even show that one serving of grape juice is as good for your heart and arteries as a daily dose of baby aspirin. So drink up!

This sweet beverage contains several powerful ingredients. Quercetin, a flavonoid found in grape skins, acts as an antioxidant to prevent LDL cholesterol from collecting on your artery walls. Resveratrol, also found in the skin, thwarts inflammation and blood clots. Meanwhile, procyanidins in the seeds help keep blood vessels relaxed and exert antioxidant powers of their own.

You've probably heard about the heart-healing powers of red wine. Because red wine uses the grape skin during processing, it boasts some of the same antioxidants as grape juice. Several European studies suggest a glass or two a day will lower your risk of dying from heart disease by about 40 percent.

If you don't drink red wine, how can you get all those eager little antioxidants to zap your nasty free radicals? Nonalcoholic wine and grape juice have about half the flavonoids of red wine but are still chock-full of antioxidants. Try substituting grape juice for your morning orange juice for a heart-healthy start to your day. Just remember that one cup of commercial, unsweetened grape juice has 154 calories. So if you're watching your weight, drink the juice but cut out another snack.

Pros and cons of drinking alcohol

There's a lot of press about the benefits of drinking — how alcoholic beverages, such as red wine, may lower your risk for angina, heart disease, and heart attack. Does that mean you should drink?

Alcohol provides lots of energy in the form of calories — remember that if you're watching your weight — but it contains few nutrients. And it may also contribute to age-related problems, like cataracts and memory loss, and can lead to nerve damage in people with diabetes.

The bottom line — weigh your health risks and discuss them with your doctor, especially if you take prescription drugs. Should you decide to drink, do so with meals and in moderation. That means no more than 12 ounces of beer or 4 ounces of wine each day for women. Men can generally double that amount. If you drink more, you cancel out any health benefits and can actually damage your heart muscles and arteries.

Southern grapes good for the heart

Most traditional Southern cooking isn't known for being heart-healthy. Gravy, fried pork chops, and buttered biscuits and grits may taste great, but they add too much fat to your diet and shoot your cholesterol higher than a Georgia pine.

The South does have at least one healthy food to contribute to the cause of good heart health – a grape known as the muscadine or scuppernong. Southern cooks have long made use of this tough-skinned but tasty fruit by making jams, preserves, juice, wine, and even muscadine hull pies. Scientists have found that this modest fruit contains substantial amounts of resveratrol, the substance in red wine believed to contribute to a healthy heart. Muscadines are high in fiber and carbohydrates but low in fat and protein.

If you don't drink wine but would like to take advantage of the heart-protecting effect of resveratrol, try some muscadine jam on your toast or try the supplement Resvinatrol Complete, containing a premium muscadine grape blend and muscadine grape seed extract. One serving of muscadine jam contains as much resveratrol as 4 ounces of red wine, and two capsules of Resvinatrol Complete contain 100 mg of resveratrol or as much as 156 glasses of red wine.

Happy 'half-hour' might help your heart

The relationship between alcohol and prevention of heart disease is one of those good news/bad news stories. What it seems to boil down to is this – if you drink alcohol in moderation, you may be able to cut your risk of a heart attack or angina in half. But if you have more than two drinks a day, your risk of high blood pressure, stroke, cancer, and many other serious health problems increases dramatically.

Moderate drinking means one to two drinks a day. If you drink more than this amount, the benefits are lost. With three or more drinks a day, the risk of death increases with each additional drink. One drink equals a 12-ounce bottle of beer, a 4-ounce glass of wine, or a 1 1/2-ounce shot of 80-proof spirits. They all contain the same amount of alcohol, one-half ounce.

Researchers think alcohol helps the heart by increasing HDL, the "good" cholesterol. HDLs remove the "bad" LDL cholesterol from the walls of the arteries and carry it back to the liver. Other research suggests alcohol also keeps blood clots from forming and may even break up blood clots as they form.

Many studies have focused on red wine and dark beer, based on the idea that antioxidants in wine and beer and not alcohol may protect the heart. Although the evidence is not conclusive, one type of alcoholic beverage doesn't seem to be better for your heart than another.

However, concentrated alcohol from distilled spirits, like whiskey, vodka, rum, gin, or brandy, can overwhelm your body's first pass metabolism. Here's what happens.

When you drink alcohol, it's absorbed by your digestive system. The alcohol is then carried to your liver before it reaches the rest of your body. The liver metabolizes the alcohol so a smaller amount enters your bloodstream. When your first pass metabolism is overwhelmed, it can cause rapidly peaking spikes in blood alcohol, as much as nine times higher than drinking the same amount of alcohol as beer or wine. Thus, drinking distilled spirits can be very damaging, even at levels that might seem moderate. The sensible conclusion is that beer and wine are better for your overall health than spirits.

Clearly, there is both good and bad to be said for alcohol use. That's why the American Heart Association has developed the following guidelines:

▸ Talk to your doctor about your personal risks and benefits. If you have a family history of alcoholism, high triglyceride level, inflammation of the pancreas, liver disease, certain blood disorders, heart failure, or uncontrolled high blood pressure, drinking alcohol could be dangerous. Pregnant women and people taking medication that interacts with alcohol should avoid drinking alcohol.

▶ If none of the above conditions exists, one or two drinks a day can be considered safe.

▶ Never operate machinery or motor vehicles when using alcohol.

▶ Discuss with your doctor the risks and benefits from time to time as part of your regular medical care. If you are having problems as a result of your drinking or you are drinking heavily, ask your doctor for guidance.

▶ Adolescents and young adults should be counseled about the risks and benefits before they develop a drinking habit.

Everyone is different, but if you follow this advice, you may reap the heart-healthy benefits from a glass of your favorite wine.

Buy the best chocolate

Dove dark chocolate may be the one brand that's actually good for your heart. Cocoapro, the cocoa in Dove dark choco-late, is specially processed to retain more flavonoids. Look for the Cocoapro logo on chocolate and consider Dove's new line of snacks, CocoVia, which contain cholesterol-fighting phyto-sterols, as well as 100 milligrams of healthy flavonoids.

A sweet way to boost good cholesterol

If it tastes good, it must be bad for you — or so you thought. New research shows that eating a small amount of dark chocolate is good for your heart. This delectable treat has something to offer besides calories — a generous helping of antioxidants called polyphenols and flavonoids, which include catechin and epicatechin.

A 1.5-ounce piece of chocolate has as many polyphenols as a glass of red wine. These antioxidants can help your heart by keeping LDL cholesterol from becoming oxidized, which can harm your arteries. A study in Finland showed the polyphenols in dark chocolate may be even better because they also raise your good cholesterol levels.

Flavonoids, on the other hand, seem to cut heart disease risk by decreasing bad LDL cholesterol and increasing good HDL cholesterol, as well as improving blood flow and lowering blood pressure. Plus, flavonoids reduce your risk of forming blood clots that lead to heart attack and stroke. Best of all, clinical studies suggest that, despite its high fat content, dark chocolate does not raise your cholesterol.

Evidence suggests you need around 125 grams – about 4.25 ounces – of flavonoid-rich chocolate daily to reap those heart-healthy antioxidant benefits. But don't eat more than one or two small bars a day. Chocolate has plenty of fat and calories – and gaining weight is bad for your heart. If you're concerned about calories, look for small pieces of dark chocolate with less fat, such as Dove's dark chocolate Promises. One piece has 42 calories and a little more than 2 grams of fat.

Unfortunately, not all chocolate is created equal. During the making of chocolate, certain processing and handling methods destroy the antioxidants. For instance, white chocolate has no flavonoids, while milk chocolate has only small amounts. Researchers also found eating milk chocolate or drinking milk with dark chocolate interferes with the absorption of antioxidants, canceling out some of their health benefits. Cocoa powder and dark chocolate seem to offer the most heart-healthy benefits.

To help keep your flavonoid levels from tapering off, eat other foods rich in the same flavonoid as chocolate, like green and black tea, sweet cherries, apples, purple grapes, blackberries, red wine, and raspberries.

Healthy, homemade chocolaty treats

Mmmm. Chocolate-dipped strawberries and homemade chocolate candy are so good — if you know what you're doing. For starters, cut semi-sweet or dark chocolate into small pieces for quick melting. Place them in the top of a double boiler, keeping the water hot but not boiling. Don't let the top pan touch the hot water in the lower pan, since that could burn the chocolate. Stir constantly to keep the heat evenly distributed.

Or use your microwave for a quick melt. Heat dark chocolate on medium at 50-percent power. Stir every 15 seconds, and remove the chocolate just before it finishes melting. Continue stirring until it has melted.

To soften hardening chocolate, add a bit of canola oil until it liquefies again. Never add water to chocolate, which is oil-based. It won't mix, and your batch will be ruined. Beware of drops of moisture on utensils and bowls that could spoil your hard work.

Chocolate products containing cocoa butter are generally healthy if consumed in moderation because of the antioxidants in chocolate. Watch out for chocolate that contains other fats, like butterfat or palm oil. These can clog your arteries.

Behold the amazing benefits of blueberries

Every now and then, a great food comes along that not only tastes good but also is good for you. Blueberries are sweet, juicy, cute, delicious, and they're packed full of all sorts of amazing health benefits — like vitamin C, fiber, calcium, and iron. As far as getting antioxidant protection, you can't do better than a serving of blueberries.

No matter how healthy you may be, molecules called free radicals are created in your body whenever cells turn oxygen into energy. These molecules are out to destroy healthy cells. Given enough time and opportunity, free radicals cause all kinds of diseases – even heart disease and cancer. Luckily, nature provides a delicious antidote in blueberries.

Each little fruit contains pigments called anthocyanins, which give the berry its blue color – kind of like dye you can eat. But anthocyanins are also potent antioxidants that hunt down and destroy free radicals. Scientists at the USDA–ARS Human Nutrition Research Center on Aging came up with a way to measure the total amount of antioxidants in foods. Blueberries scored near the top of the list. They discovered blueberries are so full of goodness that a half-cup serving has the same amount of antioxidants as five servings of peas, carrots, apples, squash, or broccoli.

Beautiful blueberries from your backyard

If you're planting blueberry bushes, why not plant at least two varieties? After all, blueberry varieties from the "rabbiteye" group won't even produce berries if you plant just one bush. They need to cross-pollinate to grow berries. In addition, the "highbush" varieties can produce berries with one bush, but you'll get better results from two highbush varieties.

Follow these tips for better berries.

▶ Blueberries are acid-loving plants. Water them with a mixture of 1 pint vinegar to 2 gallons water. Pour it around the base of the plants, not over them. Direct contact with the vinegar can cause the leaves to fall off.

▶ Old, rotting sawdust is actually a mouthwatering dessert for your blueberry plants. New sawdust just won't cut it. To please your blueberries, sawdust used as mulch needs to be old enough to rot a little. But don't use sawdust from chemically treated wood.

"Blueberries provide a relatively concentrated source of antioxidants," says Dr. Ronald L. Prior, one of the researchers. "With other fruits and vegetables, blueberries provide a way to increase antioxidant intake, which may have long-term health benefits."

You'll find members of the blueberry family throughout Europe and Asia. But more than 40 varieties are also native to North America. Don't confuse them with huckleberries, however, which look similar but have large seeds.

For years, doctors have known free radicals attack your arteries, leaving them scarred and more easily clogged by fatty deposits. The longer this process goes on, the higher your risk for heart attacks and strokes. But they also know certain antioxidants fight free-radical damage and keep your blood from getting too sticky.

German researchers discovered that people who ate the most antioxidant-rich foods, like blueberries, were the least likely to die of a heart attack. If heart disease runs in your family, blueberries, which help keep your arteries open and strong, could be one delicious way to protect yourself.

Along with battling heart disease, blueberries do some other great things for your body.

▶ Put the crunch on cancer. Cancer is often the result of free radicals gone haywire. But you can short-circuit these killers with powerful antioxidants like the ones found in blueberries. Studies in Germany found foods high in antioxidants, like anthocyanins, seemed to protect people from cancer.

▶ Stabilize blood sugar. Blueberries are a favorite folk remedy for high blood sugar, but scientists only recently found proof. Animal studies in Italy showed blueberries lowered blood sugar levels by about 26 percent. Although diabetes is a serious illness that requires professional care, it certainly couldn't hurt to sprinkle a handful of these healthy berries on your cereal. If you have diabetes, talk to your doctor before you change your diet.

▶ Give UTIs the slip. Researchers know *E. coli* bacteria cause some urinary tract infections (UTIs). For years, doctors thought the acid in certain fruits, especially cranberries, worked to get rid of UTIs by chasing away these bacteria. Now they know blueberries, like cranberries, contain antioxidants that actually change the structure of the bacteria – they become powerless to attach themselves to your cells.

▶ Keep your mind sharp. Exciting new studies at Tufts University in Boston suggest blueberry extract may improve memory, coordination, and speed tests.

▶ Restore regularity. People in Sweden have used blueberries for hundreds of years as a cure for diarrhea. It may be blueberries counteract the bacteria that cause diarrhea, or it could be their soluble fiber keeps your bowels humming along regularly. A single cup of blueberries contains about 15 percent of your daily recommended intake of fiber.

Resolve the fresh vs. frozen fruit debate

You've always heard that fresh fruits are better than frozen, canned, or dried fruits, but that may not necessarily be true.

Truth is, frozen and canned fruits generally have the same nutritional value as their fresh relatives. In some cases, they may even be healthier. Canned peaches, for instance, have only one-thousandth of the pesticides found on fresh peaches, possibly because they're peeled before processing. Just remember, to get the same benefits from canned fruit, you must buy the kind packed in its own juice, not in calorie-laden syrup.

Dried fruits also have the same nutrition as their fresh siblings, but dried fruits also tend to have more sugar.

Careful cooking tames heart villain

Sometimes how you cook is more important than what you cook. Chemicals called advanced glycation end products (AGEs) are to blame. These components form naturally when foods containing sugars, fats, and proteins are cooked at high temperatures for a long time.

Scientists have known about AGEs for a while, but they only recently discovered the danger to people with diabetes. Recent research shows AGEs could be a major reason why people with diabetes are at high risk for heart disease. The researchers suspect AGEs cause overreaction of the immune system of a person with diabetes. This change could damage blood vessels.

But you can control AGEs in your diet.

▶ Limit animal foods, including meat, cheese, and egg yolks, which can be high in AGEs after cooking.

▶ Use high-humidity cooking methods, like boiling and steaming, or stir-frying to produce fewer AGEs. Avoid baking, grilling, and broiling.

Tiny fruit puts the squeeze on plaque

This fruit can promote weight loss, lower cholesterol, improve insulin levels, and heal fatty livers – even while on a high-fat diet. Not only are cherries deliciously sweet, they're a sweet deal for your heart.

In a new lab study, researchers at Michigan State University put some mice on a high-fat diet and others on a low-fat diet. The high-fat mice quickly gained weight, developed fatty livers, and became glucose intolerant. Researchers then began feeding them anthocyanins, antioxidant compounds that give cherries their red color, in addition to their fatty food. After eight weeks, these obese, glucose-intolerant mice had lost weight, lowered their cholesterol, raised their insulin levels, were more glucose-sensitive, and once again had healthy livers.

Antioxidants are like guests at a party – the more the merrier. Cherries pack no less than 17 powerful antioxidant compounds that clear away artery-clogging plaque far better than vitamin supplements. These compounds have even more antioxidant activity than heavyweights like vitamin C or vitamin E supplements.

These antioxidants may protect against atherosclerosis and heart disease by preventing the buildup of plaque in your arteries. Anthocyanins also squash inflammation, which can contribute to atherosclerosis. They work by stopping the enzymes that make prostaglandins, hormone-like substances that cause inflammation and pain.

Cherries also provide fiber and potassium, two winning warriors in the battle against heart disease. Fiber lowers cholesterol and reduces your risk of heart disease and stroke. Potassium, too, shields you from stroke. It also fights heart disease by controlling your blood pressure so your heart doesn't have to work overtime.

Researchers in the rat study used Cornelian cherries, but they say the more popular tart cherries are similar. So whether you enjoy them dried, jammed, or straight off the stem, give cherries a try.

Take a bite out of plaque buildup

Whether you like a tangy marinara sauce or a luscious beefsteak tomato fresh off the vine, you may be on the right track to prevent a heart attack.

The French once called tomatoes "love apples." Turns out, that's appropriate because researchers think tomatoes may help prevent heart trouble. In fact, the juice from this artery-cleaning vegetable acts like a scrub brush to clear out cholesterol and reduce high blood pressure.

The trouble starts when LDL cholesterol in your blood becomes oxidized. "When LDL is oxidized, it leads to the formation of plaque in the vessel — known as atherosclerosis," explains Dr. Joye Willcox, a registered dietician and owner of the private weight management practice Healthy Diets, Inc. As more plaques form, the walls of your arteries become thicker, constricting the flow of blood. Eventually, an artery may get clogged enough to cause a heart attack. But that doesn't have to happen.

Willcox and other scientists think something special in tomatoes may help prevent plaque. The most likely candidates may be antioxidants. "Antioxidants provide protection in the inner layer of blood vessels to prevent LDL cholesterol from being oxidized," says Willcox.

That may mean something as convenient as tomato juice could stop your cholesterol from oxidizing and sticking to your artery walls. You may be able to stop plaque and clogged arteries before they can even get started.

Get the facts. Some studies suggest the tomato's most famous antioxidant — lycopene — could be the hero that rescues hearts.

▸ Dutch researchers examined the blood vessels and blood of 108 elderly people. The higher the amount of lycopene they found in a person's blood, the lower the risk of atherosclerosis seemed to be — especially for smokers or former smokers.

▸ A study of more than 1,000 men in Finland found those with low levels of lycopene in their blood had thicker artery walls — a sign of atherosclerosis.

▸ According to American research, older women with more lycopene in their blood may have up to 34 percent less risk of heart disease than those with the lowest lycopene levels.

Choose foods, not supplements. Willcox and her colleagues examined the research on what lycopene can do without help from other nutrients. They found some studies where lycopene reduced LDL oxidation and others where it did not. Even studies on other tomato antioxidants had the same mixed results. Yet, research on whole fruits and vegetables consistently showed more promise.

Tomatoes aren't one-trick ponies. Lycopene may get the most attention, but these mouth-watering vegetables contain an army of nutrients. Their folate cleans up homocysteine, an amino acid that links with cholesterol to give your heart double trouble. Plus, they're chock-full of potassium, a mineral crucial for lowering blood pressure. Willcox and her colleagues concluded that eating tomatoes and tomato products could be good protection for your heart.

Cook for a healthier heart. "One cup of tomato sauce or two cups of tomato juice would provide approximately 40 milligrams of lycopene," Willcox says. That amount of daily lycopene from food may be enough to affect the oxidation of LDL cholesterol, according to one study. Another study suggested that drinking 17 ounces of tomato juice every day could do your heart good. But you can also eat your way to lower heart attack risk.

"Cooking appears to increase the absorption of lycopene," says Willcox. That means you may get more lycopene from processed tomato products – especially those with a little oil, which helps your body take in more lycopene. For best results, stick with healthy oils, like olive oil, and avoid saturated fats and trans fats.

Tomatoes aren't for everyone. If you have heartburn or acid reflux, tomatoes could make your discomfort worse. Some experts also suspect tomatoes may aggravate arthritis, so talk to your doctor if you're concerned.

Yummy spice cuts cholesterol and blood sugar

It controls blood sugar, cuts triglycerides, even lowers "bad" cholesterol. It's not a drug – it's a spice, and it's probably in your pantry right now.

A spoonful of sugar helps the medicine go down — but a spoonful of cinnamon does much, much more. Well known as a tasty addition to buns and apple pies, it gave diabetes researchers a big surprise when it succeeded in lowering blood sugar just as well as the nutrient they were studying.

The active ingredient in cinnamon, a polyphenol compound called methylhydroxy chalcone polymer (MHCP), acts like insulin in your body. Insulin helps control blood sugar levels, but it also plays a part regulating triglyceride and cholesterol levels. That may explain why diabetics tend to have higher cholesterol and triglycerides in addition to higher blood sugar than most people. Cinnamon appears to lower blood sugar along with LDL cholesterol and triglycerides. Diabetics also tend to have high amounts of free radicals circulating in their bodies. Lab experiments showed cinnamon effectively neutralized these damaging molecules.

The strongest evidence for cinnamon comes from a recent Pakistani study of 30 men and 30 women with diabetes. People in the study took either 1 gram, 3 grams, or 6 grams of cinnamon, in the form of cinnamon capsules, each day for 40 days. Other study participants took equivalent amounts of placebo or fake pill. People taking cinnamon, regardless of the dose, saw several significant improvements.

▸ Fasting blood sugar dropped 18 to 29 percent.

▸ Total cholesterol levels fell 12 to 26 percent, while LDL cholesterol decreased by 7 to 27 percent.

▸ Triglyceride levels plummeted by 23 to 30 percent.

Plus, the positive effects linger. Even 20 days after stopping cinnamon treatment, people often maintained lower blood sugar, cholesterol, and triglyceride levels.

What's more, a little dab may do it. People in studies benefited from taking just 1 gram — about half a teaspoon — of cinnamon each day. Don't miss out on this super spice. Sprinkle cinnamon on oatmeal, cereal, toast, yogurt, apples, and other fruit; spice up cooked carrots, squash, sweet potatoes, and meats; or stir hot drinks with cinnamon sticks instead of a spoon. Never eat cinnamon oil, which can be poisonous even in small amounts.

Pick the perfect seasoning

Check out these creative salt alternatives for spicing up your meals, courtesy of the American Heart Association. Experiment with new flavors. Your heart and your taste buds will thank you.'

fish	basil, curry powder, dill, garlic, lemon juice, dry mustard, nutmeg, paprika, parsley, sage, or turmeric
chicken	curry powder, dill, ginger, dry mustard, nutmeg, or rosemary
lean meats	allspice, bay leaves, caraway seeds, chives, curry powder, garlic, lemon juice, dry mustard, onion, paprika, parsley, sage, thyme, or turmeric
soups	basil, bay leaves, caraway seeds, chives, dill, garlic, onions, paprika, parsley, or thyme
stews	allspice, basil, bay leaves, caraway seeds, or sage
sauces	basil, chives, cider vinegar, dry mustard, paprika, parsley, rosemary, thyme, or turmeric
vegetables	chives, cider vinegar, garlic, lemon juice, onion, paprika, or parsley

Shake your taste for salt

Salt looks harmless, but don't let its innocent appearance fool you. Higher salt intake means higher blood pressure. That's because salt causes your body to retain water, increasing the amount of blood in your arteries. It also causes small arteries to constrict, making it harder for blood to squeeze through.

Some people are more sensitive to salt than others. In fact, about half the U.S. population is salt-sensitive. For these people, reducing salt intake drastically lowers blood pressure. Those who fall in this category, according to a recent analysis of the Dietary Approaches to Stop Hypertension (DASH)-Sodium Trial, include people with high blood pressure, blacks, women, and people older than age 45.

Because it's hard to test for salt sensitivity, the National Heart, Lung, and Blood Institute recommends everyone cut back. Right now, the average American consumes more than 4,000 milligrams (mg) of sodium daily. However, people should limit sodium to 2,300 mg a day — roughly equal to one teaspoon of salt. If you have high blood pressure, you should cut that down to 1,500 mg or less.

If your blood pressure is fine, you probably don't worry about salt intake. Think again. High blood pressure raises your stroke risk, but so can blood pressure in the upper ranges of "normal," say British researchers. They found older adults cut their risk of stroke by eating less salt, even if they didn't have high blood pressure. How? Lowering your salt intake may lead to a drop in blood pressure, even if your pressure is usually normal. This, in turn, can reduce your stroke risk.

Need another reason to shake your salt craving? When you eat too much of it, your kidneys work especially hard to flush it out — and they often end up flushing out other important minerals, like calcium. What's more, calcium and salt compete in a race to get absorbed by your body. Sometimes extra salt wins and calcium passes right on out through your urine.

All this calcium loss can contribute to osteoporosis. In fact, if you have thinning bones, you may have heart disease, too. At least in women, low bone density appears to go hand in hand with hardening of the arteries. Fighting one disease by slashing salt intake may help you beat the other.

Spice up your life without salt

Won't your food taste bland without salt? Not if you make some smart — and delicious — substitutions. For instance, garlic and onions do more than just add flavor to food. Sulfur compounds in both fight poor circulation by keeping blood platelets from clumping together and making your blood sticky.

Quercetin and other flavonoids in onions also help stop LDL cholesterol from oxidizing and blocking your arteries. While recent studies aren't as conclusive regarding garlic's heart-protective powers, it still adds flavor without contributing to high blood pressure.

Lemon, lime, vinegar, and many herbs and spices give your food amazing flavor without the danger that comes with salt. As an added bonus, some seasonings are packed with heart-protecting antioxidants. Try ground cloves, ground cinnamon, and oregano for the most antioxidant punch.

Spot hidden sources of salt

Just laying off the saltshaker won't solve the problem of too much sodium. Most of it hides in prepared foods and packaged foods, so it's hard to know how much salt you're getting.

For instance, you may think coffee is bad for your blood pressure, but drinking sodas may be worse. In fact, having too much of this everyday drink could be what's raising your blood pressure, since a single 12-ounce can contains about 50 milligrams of sodium. Here's how most people divvy up their daily salt.

▶ 10 percent comes from salt naturally found in foods

▶ 15 percent comes from table salt added during cooking or at the table

▶ 75 percent comes from salt added to pre-packaged foods during processing

As you can see, processed foods, such as frozen dinners, restaurant meals, and canned foods, contribute the most salt in your diet. If you cut back on them and limit the salt you use while cooking and at the table, you'll be on your way to lower blood pressure.

Load up on fruits and veggies. In their natural, fresh form, they're low in sodium and packed with potassium, a mineral that may help reduce blood pressure.

Buy fresh or frozen fish, poultry, and meat. These tend to have less salt than their canned and processed counterparts. The exceptions are cured meats, like bacon and ham, which are usually loaded with salt. Whenever possible, avoid processed meats, like cold cuts. And if something is labeled "pickled" or "cured," that means it's been soaked in salt, and you should avoid it. Even those oh-so-convenient rotisserie chickens in your grocery store are pre-treated with salt.

Go easy on the sides. A lot of salt in your diet comes from condiments, like ketchup, mustard, steak and soy sauce, and extras like pickles. Would you believe a large dill pickle contains over 1,000 mg of salt? Munch on carrot sticks with your lunch, instead. Skip the high-sodium cup of soup with your sandwich, and try a side of vegetables or a salad. Treat even low-sodium versions of soy and teriyaki sauces like salt, and use them sparingly.

Do it yourself. Your best bet is to cut back on restaurant meals and processed foods, like cold cuts, canned vegetables and soups, broths, frozen dinners, instant rice and pasta mixes, cheeses, salad dressings, snack foods, and fast foods. When you prepare your own meals from scratch, it's harder for salt to sneak up on you.

Be stingy. When you cook, try using half the salt called for in the recipe. It might be possible to cut salt completely from some recipes.

You can always add a bit at the table. Just don't salt your food automatically, like many people do. At least taste food first, and if you feel it needs a little something, try pepper, onion or garlic powder, or a salt-free commercial product, like Mrs. Dash or Spike.

Wash away salt. You can cut the sodium in canned vegetables up to 40 percent just by rinsing them with water before you eat them.

Read labels. If you want to avoid heart disease, you'll have to check nutrition labels carefully for sodium content and change the way you eat. Products low in sodium often advertise that fact. Look for items marked "no salt added," "low sodium," or "reduced sodium." Check the Nutrition Facts label, too, and look for foods with less than 5 percent – about 120 mg – of your maximum daily sodium allowance.

Drink plenty of water. It's generally low in salt and helps flush any excess out of your body. Check the labels on bottled water for their sodium content.

Ask before you order. Eating out can be a challenge when you're on a special diet. Ask your waiter if the food you're ordering is prepared with salt or MSG, which is high in sodium. Many restaurants are able to cook your food the way you want it. Order sauces on the side and use them sparingly, or not at all, if they're salty.

Sodium content of common foods

Cutting back on sodium is crucial to lowering your blood pressure. That means reading labels carefully. Food manufacturers know people like salt. That's why they've been slow to cut back, thinking you won't buy their food if it tastes a little different. Nearly a third of the sodium you eat likely comes from baked goods and cereal. Foods made from milk also tend to be high in salt. Fast food is even worse. A Big Mac and large fries roughly packs a whopping 1,500 milligrams (mg) of sodium.

When it comes to cutting sodium, your motto should be "fresh is best." Need more convincing? Here's a look at how much salt is hiding in your food.

Food	Sodium (milligrams)
Meats	
3 oz cooked roast beef	53
3 oz cooked chicken	50
1 large hot dog	638
3 oz chipped beef	2,953
1 package Oscar Mayer Lunchables Deluxe Turkey & Ham with Swiss & Cheddar	1,940
1 package Swanson's Hungry Man XXL Roasted Carved Turkey	5,410
Vegetables	
1/2 cup cooked carrots	50
1 small baked potato	20
1 cooked ear of corn	3
1 cup creamed corn	572
Fruits	
1 peach	0
1 cup canned peaches	16
1 slice peach pie	253
1 apple	0
1 slice apple pie	444
Assorted store-bought goods	
plain bagel	379
5 medium pretzel twists	486
1/2 cup low-fat cottage cheese	459
1 tablespoon La Choy soy sauce	1,260
Fast food and restaurant meals	
fish sandwich	615
small cheeseburger	725
1 serving onion rings	800
roast beef sandwich	792

Food	Sodium (milligrams)
Reuben sandwich	3,270
egg and bacon biscuit	999
baked potato with cheese sauce and chili	701
chocolate shake	273
cheese fries with ranch dressing	4,890
General Tso's chicken with rice	3,150
spaghetti with sausage	2,440
Frozen foods and dinners	
TV dinner – chicken, corn, mashed potatoes, and chocolate pudding	1,820
Stouffer's Slow Roasted Beef & Gravy Homestyle Dinner	1,510
Banquet Macaroni & Cheese Dinner	1,500

Eat less sodium to keep more calcium

It's a major mineral in salt and a major enemy to your heart. While some foods naturally contain small amounts of sodium, most of it is added during cooking or processing to boost flavor. Salt lends a hand in regulating your body fluids and blood pressure, and it helps muscles and nerves work properly. You only need a tiny bit of sodium to get these jobs done – about 600 milligrams (mg) or less than one-fourth teaspoon of salt.

Most people, however, get over 3,000 mg of sodium daily. If you eat too much salt, your kidneys, which regulate the mineral and water balance in your body, must work harder to flush out the extra sodium. Unfortunately, many other important minerals, like calcium, get flushed out as well. The more salt you eat, the more calcium you lose. The more calcium you lose, the greater your bone loss and your risk for osteoporosis.

Limiting your sodium to less than 2,400 mg a day – about one teaspoon of salt – could not only slow down this calcium loss but also put a lid on high blood pressure. People who are salt-sensitive and already have high blood pressure could especially benefit from eating less salt.

Naturally, the best way to cut back sodium is to limit salt and salty foods. If you're a snacker, you may find that especially difficult. Read the Nutrition Facts label on foods to discover the sodium content.

Salt substitute could save your life

Potassium-enriched salt substitutes are nothing new, but a new study from Taiwan suggests they could save your life. Doctors sometimes advise people with high blood pressure to switch to a salt substitute made with potassium, which cuts the amount of salt you add to your food and gives you a dose of blood pressure-lowering potassium.

That could be a big deal if you're at risk of heart problems. Past studies suggest getting more potassium in your diet could drop high blood pressure and slash your risk of stroke death by 40 percent. Now new research shows using a salt substitute made with half potassium chloride and half sodium chloride (salt) could reduce deaths from heart disease, diabetes, high blood pressure, and stroke.

For two-and-a-half years, more than 750 elderly men in Taiwan used this potassium-enriched salt in place of regular salt. In the end, they were 40 percent less likely to die from heart disease-related ill- nesses, including stroke, diabetes, and high blood pressure than the 1,200 men using regular salt. They also lived longer and spent about 40 percent less on heart-related hospital bills.

Researchers say the benefits mostly come from getting more potassi- um, although cutting back on sodium also helped. But take note – these men did not simply add a dash of potassium-salt on top of their regular salt. They used it to replace their regular salt for a double-whammy, boosting their potassium levels while reducing their sodium intake.

Keep in mind that potassium can be harmful in large amounts, particularly if you have kidney problems or if you are taking med- ication for heart failure or high blood pressure. Talk to your doctor if you fit this description, or if you start experiencing nausea, diarrhea, weakness, or an irregular heartbeat after you begin using a potassium-enriched salt substitute.

Great idea for salt lovers

Morton Lite Salt, available at your local grocery store, is a smart way to add a little zip to your food. It contains 50-percent less sodium than regular salt and is a good source of potassium. You can use it for baking and cooking, as well as seasoning your food at the table. However, if you are on a sodium- or potassium-restricted diet or a potassium-sparing diuretic, ask your doctor for his advice before trying this product.

DASH high blood pressure in 6 simple steps

If you want to make big improvements in your blood pressure without resorting to drugs, Dietary Approaches to Stop Hypertension (DASH) could be your dream diet.

Three major studies – DASH, DASH-Sodium, and PREMIER – have proven that a diet rich in wholesome plant foods and low in salt can do just that. Best of all, the results show this diet could work for almost everyone – men and women, young people and seniors, white and black, overweight and normal weight, physically active and sedentary, and even those who don't yet have high blood pressure.

The DASH diet is built on fruits, vegetables, whole grains, and low-fat dairy products and limited in fat and refined carbohydrates. Nutritionist Mary Beth Horrell, with the Diabetes and Health Education Center at Asheville, North Carolina's Mission Hospital, can vouch for the healthfulness of the DASH diet. Her hospital's high blood pressure program has used it for years.

When the DASH plan was first investigated, Horrell says, it emphasized limiting fats and sweets and eating well-rounded, nutritious meals. Those who used it saw their blood pressure drop. Then DASH research began to focus on sodium, and blood pressure numbers fell even further. "The final conclusion," says Horrell, "was that both approaches are effective independently, but when combined they have the most beneficial results."

What's especially exciting is the fact that DASH can lower blood pressure as much as any single blood-pressure medication can — 10, 14, even 16 points or more. In the DASH-Sodium study, about 400 people tried several combinations of diets and salt levels to see which worked best. Those who experienced the biggest improvement in their blood pressure were people who followed the DASH eating plan and cut back their sodium to approximately 1,200 milligrams (mg) a day. It's not as hard as it sounds. Reducing sodium isn't merely a matter of throwing the salt shaker away, Horrell says. "DASH is inherently lower in sodium because it emphasizes fresh fruits and vegetables, which have very little sodium." And the results may be worth it, especially for people over age 45 who benefited the most from lowering their sodium.

There's more good news. Researchers think sticking to a low-sodium diet could keep reducing your blood pressure over the course of your lifetime. Even if your pressure only drops a little, experts believe following the DASH-Sodium diet long-term could protect you from the slow rise in blood pressure that often comes with age, thus lowering your risk for heart-related death. Check out these basic tips to start putting the lid on high blood pressure. These serving recommendations are based on a 2,000-calorie-a-day diet.

▶ Learn to love whole grains. Whole grains provided up to half the fiber, protein, calcium, magnesium, potassium, folate, and zinc that people in the DASH-Sodium study ate. To reach similar goals, eat seven to eight servings of whole grain-products — not refined — every day.

155

▶ Fill up on fresh fruit. Fruits are an excellent source of potassium, a mineral that may help control your blood pressure. Eating at least four to five servings daily will help you get the large amounts of potassium prescribed by the DASH diet.

▶ Munch on more vegetables. Strive for four to five servings of vegetables each day. They provide about 15 percent of the magnesium, potassium, and calcium you get on the DASH diet, and they're terrific sources of fiber, folate, and vitamins A, C, and E.

▶ Develop a taste for dairy. Make two to three servings part of your daily plan. Just be sure you choose low-fat products.

▶ Eat fish, poultry, and other meats sparingly. Under the DASH plan, you should limit these meats to no more than two servings a day. Make a point of choosing fish and poultry more often than red meat and treat them as one part of your meal, not the main course.

▶ Add a few legumes, nuts, and seeds. They deliver even more of the nutrients important to DASH, like protein, potassium, magnesium, and fiber. Serve up four to five servings of legumes a week, along with a handful of nuts or seeds for a tasty snack.

People who eat a typical American diet get most of their energy from refined grains, fats, sweets, and oils. On the DASH diet, however, your energy comes from more heart friendly whole grains, fruits, and low-fat dairy products. This diet also gives you more vitamins, thanks to all those extra fruits and vegetables.

Horrell believes the DASH plan is here to stay — it works and focuses on moderation. "It doesn't eliminate any food groups. It includes foods that anybody has access to. It's satisfying nutritionally. And people who use it aren't hungry. There aren't any dangers associated with DASH that I'm aware of. DASH makes sense to me."

You can also order a copy of *Your Guide to Lowering Your Blood Pressure with DASH*. This pamphlet from the National Heart, Lung, and Blood Institute contains sample menus and details about the original DASH diet study. Just call their Health Information Center at 301-592-8563 or visit them on the Internet at *http://emall.nhlbihin.net*.

Talk to your doctor before making any major changes to your eating habits. Keep taking your blood pressure medicine, and don't tamper with your dosage without first consulting your doctor. If you slip up and overindulge in unhealthy foods, don't give up — for your blood pressure's sake.

DASH at a glance

These serving guidelines give you a quick snapshot of the DASH diet. Yet, they aren't the whole story. Remember, you also need to limit your sodium to 1,200 milligrams per day, plus trim saturated fat and cholesterol from your daily food choices.

Food group	Daily servings
grains and grain products	7 – 8
vegetables	4 – 5
fruits	4 – 5
dairy (low-fat or fat free)	2 – 3
fats and oils	2 – 3
meats, poultry, and fish	2 or less
nuts, seeds, and dry beans	4 – 5 per week
sweets	5 per week

Spot foods that lead to blood sugar spikes

Certain foods can cause your blood sugar to soar – and increase your risk of heart disease. Use this handy chart to help you avoid foods that are dangerous to people who have diabetes. You don't have to eliminate these foods from your diet, but you may want to eat them sparingly.

bagels	bread stuffing
Kellogg's Corn Flakes cereal	Kellogg's Crispix cereal
Nabisco Corn Chex cereal	Nabisco Rice Chex cereal
cheese curls	instant Cream of Wheat
dried dates	dinner rolls
french fries	fruit punch
Gatorade sports drink	graham crackers
jellybeans	kaiser rolls
licorice	Melba toast
parsnips	popcorn
russet potatoes	pretzels
most rice, except brown rice	rice cakes
scones	soda crackers
waffles	white bread

Think like Popeye to K.O. high blood pressure

Three's a crowd – except when it comes to fighting high blood pressure. That's when you need the triple threat of potassium, magnesium, and calcium, not to mention the powerful B-vitamin sidekicks.

Popeye knew a thing or two about the super powers of spinach. Gobbling some spinach may not give you the strength of 10 men, but it sure gives your heart a big boost. This tasty and popular food is naturally low in sodium, saturated fat, and cholesterol. Plus, it's chock full of potassium, magnesium, and calcium, not to mention the B vitamins that nix heart disease and keep your brain chemicals in balance.

Pile on the potassium. If you're battling high blood pressure, you probably know all about the perils of salt. But potassium plays just as big a role in capping your blood pressure. This vital mineral neutralizes sodium by flushing it out in your urine. It also relaxes your blood vessels, which improves blood flow.

Study after study shows that adding potassium to your diet helps lower blood pressure. Limit your salt for an even greater effect. People with high blood pressure benefit the most from this strategy, but you may see improvement even if you're in the normal range.

And that's not all. This miracle mineral boasts at least seven other heart-healthy benefits, including these:

▶ protects your blood vessels from damage

▶ prevents dangerous irregular heartbeats

▶ reduces your risk of stroke

▶ widens blood vessels

▶ suppresses renin, an enzyme produced by your kidneys that contributes to high blood pressure

▶ prompts your sympathetic nervous system to regulate your blood pressure

▶ prods your kidneys to get rid of more sodium and less calcium through your urine

It's easy to boost your potassium intake. Just eat a cup of cooked spinach or a side of fresh spinach salad. This leafy green is one of the most potassium-rich foods you can eat. Other good sources include peas, beans, apricots, peaches, bananas, prunes, oranges, stewed tomatoes, sweet potatoes, avocados, and figs.

Maximize your magnesium. Consider magnesium one of potassium's sidekicks in the fight against high blood pressure. This mineral relaxes blood vessels and balances the amount of sodium and potassium in your blood cells – less sodium, more potassium.

A four-year study of more than 30,000 men found that getting more magnesium into your diet was significantly associated with a lower risk of high blood pressure. In fact, the Joint National Committee on Prevention, Detection, Evaluation, and Treatment of High Blood Pressure recommends maintaining an adequate magnesium intake as a way to prevent and manage high blood pressure.

Spinach, beans, nuts, and seeds are packed with this mineral, as are whole-wheat breads and cereals, broccoli, chard, okra, oysters, scallops, sea bass, and mackerel.

Cram in the calcium. As you get older, your systolic blood pressure, the top number in a blood pressure reading, tends to go up. A recent University of South Carolina study found that boosting your calcium intake may help slow this increase.

Calcium helps control blood pressure by helping your body get rid of sodium through your urine. In fact, people who get very little calcium in their diet often have high blood pressure. But if you think dairy products are the only way to boost your calcium, think again. A cup of cooked spinach contains an amazing 24 percent of your daily calcium. Broccoli, turnip greens, and canned salmon with bones are other good, nondairy sources.

Fight back with folate. Researchers found that an amino acid called homocysteine pairs up with cholesterol to damage your arteries, which can cause a heart attack or stroke. Plus, high levels of homocysteine in your blood make you more likely to develop heart disease.

Luckily, you can battle back. The B vitamins folate and B6 help convert homocysteine into a less-dangerous substance. Spinach is a top-notch source of both these B's.

You may do your brain a favor, too. High rates of depression are also linked to a lack of vitamin B6 and thiamin, another B-vitamin spinach boasts in high amounts. B6 helps balance certain brain chemicals, keeping your emotions on an even keel, and thiamin helps nerve signals travel from your brain to other parts of your body.

Asparagus, beets, pinto beans, lentils, and enriched cereals are more good sources of folate, while bananas, chicken breast, and sweet and white potatoes are bursting with B6. For an extra dose of thiamin, look to whole grain foods and legumes, like black beans.

Discover multi-talented spinach

Spinach is packed with heart-healthy nutrients. Here's what you get from a cup of unsalted, boiled spinach

Nutrient	Percent of Daily Value (DV)	Amount
folate	66	263 mcg
magnesium	39	157 mg
calcium	24	245 mg
potassium	24	839 mg
thiamin	11	0.2 mg

Pour yourself a cup of heart health

Your morning coffee habit may do more good than just help you wake up. It may also help your heart. A recent study found drinking one to three cups of coffee a day might help protect you from heart disease. That's because coffee, rich in antioxidants, fights inflammation, which plays a major role in the development of heart disease. This stands in contrast to a previous study, which found that life-long caffeine consumption might contribute to heart disease. But coffee is not for everyone. Follow these tips to ensure safe sipping.

Keep it filtered. The type of coffee you drink may make a difference. Drinking filtered coffee does not appear to boost your risk of heart disease, even if you drink six cups or more a day. However, unfiltered or boiled coffee, such as the kind you make with a French press, may be harmful because it contains substances that raise cholesterol levels.

Beware of uncomfortable symptoms. Coffee may also be dangerous if your body metabolizes it slowly. Because of an inherited trait, some people break down coffee slower than others. Unfortunately, this trait puts you at much greater risk for a heart attack. If coffee makes you feel weak or lightheaded, quickens your pulse, or causes pain in your chest, don't drink it.

Wait before exercising. Drinking coffee right before exercising may cause problems because it narrows your blood vessels, which decreases blood flow through the arteries supplying oxygen to your heart. If you start your day with a cup of coffee, wait at least an hour before exercising.

Stay alert to a fast heartbeat. If you suffer from tachycardia, a heart rhythm problem in which your heart tends to beat too fast, you may need to cut down on the caffeine in coffee. Caffeine stimulates your heart and can cause palpitations and tachycardia. If rapid heartbeat is a problem for you, it's better to stay away from the caffeine in coffee, tea, and cola drinks.

Good news for coffee drinkers

If you need a cup of coffee to get going in the morning, here's some good news. Coffee boosts blood pressure in the short run, but regular coffee drinking does not seem to have an effect on developing high blood pressure. However, if you already have high blood pressure, you may want to limit your coffee consumption. Other beverages that may raise your blood pressure include beer, wine, and colas — including diet colas.

Reverse heart disease by this time next year

Can it really be done? Dr. Dean Ornish testified to the U.S. Senate that his program had shown some reversal of coronary artery plaque buildup after one year – and even more after five years.

Ornish is the author of *Dr. Dean Ornish's Program for Reversing Heart Disease*, a lifestyle program that advocates daily aerobic exercise; daily stress reduction; and a very low-fat, vegetarian diet. Ornish is more extreme than either the DASH or Step diets, but the results could save your life.

"The program has proven to improve blood flow to the heart by promoting plaque regression," says Jennifer Grana, a registered dietician with Highmark, Inc., who helps oversee the Ornish program in Pennsylvania hospitals. In participants in the Ornish program, this is measured by decreased chest pain and improvement in stress tests, she says.

Find out if this highly effective, all-natural treatment can flush plaque and fatty buildup out of your arteries, too.

Understand how it works. Blood clots, clogged arteries, constricted arteries, or artery spasms can limit blood flow to the heart and could trigger a heart attack. The Ornish program might help prevent these heart attack triggers.

Too much cholesterol in your blood encourages artery-clogging deposits to build up. Your "bad" LDL cholesterol level can skyrocket if your diet is high in saturated fat and cholesterol. Fortunately, your liver cells have LDL receptors that can bind and remove cholesterol, and "good" HDL cholesterol helps purge LDL, too. But they often can't work fast enough to beat the LDL overload from a poor diet. Under Ornish's program, you eat so little cholesterol and fat that your body might never have more LDL than it can eliminate.

But that's not all. Stress causes your body to release adrenaline and other hormones that increase your heart rate and raise your blood pressure, which can cause constrictions or spasms in your arteries. "There's a lot of research out there, too, that shows that hostility, isolation, and depression actually contribute to heart disease," says Grana. Both stress management and exercise help lower blood pressure, but exercise also helps promote weight loss and improve blood flow to your heart.

These guidelines summarize the Ornish program.

▶ no more than 10 percent of total calories from fat and only 5 milligrams of cholesterol per day

▶ plenty of fiber and plant foods, like fruits, vegetables, grains, and legumes

▶ little alcohol and no caffeine

▶ no oils or animal products, except nonfat milk, yogurt, and egg whites

▶ minimal salt and sugar

▶ moderate daily aerobic exercise

▶ stress-management training

▶ group support meetings

▶ no smoking

Experience amazing results. Is it possible to reverse heart disease naturally in 365 days or less? Ornish's research suggests the answer might be yes. In eight out of every 10 people studied, the arteries that had been clogged were cleaner, according to one research project.

In addition, an early test of the Ornish program found that in only 24 days participants experienced these amazing results.

▶ reduced chest pain by 91 percent

▶ improved ability to exercise

▶ reduced cholesterol levels by 21 percent

▶ lessened anxiety, fear, and depression

But there's more good news about this drug-free remedy. In three research studies, Ornish had to decrease or discontinue blood pressure medications for most participants. Their diet and lifestyle changes had brought down their blood pressure naturally. If you or someone you know has high blood pressure, this drug-free remedy could be worth checking out.

Ornish's latest research included 440 participants across the country. As with previous studies, the participants lowered LDL cholesterol, weight, and blood pressure and increased their ability to exercise. Their triglyceride levels didn't change, and their HDL cholesterol dropped but returned to starting levels by the study's end.

But Ornish's exciting research results are from people who did more than just use the diet. "The stress management, exercise, and group support are certainly extremely effective in the fight against heart disease and the goal to reverse it," says Grana.

Get expert advice. Talk with your doctor before you try the Ornish program. It isn't right for everyone. The Ornish diet is very strict, so plan ahead. You might have a hard time cutting meat and fats, including olive oil, and avoiding sugar and salt.

Getting enough fresh, unprocessed foods will be a challenge in today's on-the-go society. You must also watch your nutrient intake to make sure you don't become deficient in calcium or vitamins E, B12, and D. And eat a variety of vegetarian protein sources — like rice with beans — to meet your body's amino acid requirements. Finally, allow several hours for exercise and stress management every week. To find out more, call 800-879-2217 if you're in West Virginia or Pennsylvania — or 800-775-7674 if you live in other states.

Get the facts on low-fat eating plans

Most eating programs supported by the American Heart Association (AHA) recommend a total fat intake of no more than 20 to 35 percent of total calories. But the AHA does not recommend diets with less than 15 percent of fat from calories because short-term studies suggest these diets can raise triglycerides and reduce HDL cholesterol. No long-term studies have examined the safety and effectiveness of these very-low-fat diets.

Forbidden food actually blocks cholesterol

Surprise! When it comes to battling high cholesterol, some "evil" foods might not be villains after all. One food with a bad reputation is eggs, known for their high cholesterol content. Perhaps you've been avoiding eggs because you're worried about your cholesterol. You must be "yolking." The American Heart Association says you can enjoy several eggs a week regardless of your cholesterol level. How many eggs does that add up to?

Studies show that eating up to one egg a day does not put you at greater risk for a heart attack or stroke, although an increase in heart disease risk was seen in people with diabetes. Eggs do have lots of cholesterol, but they also provide healthy nutrients – folate and other B vitamins; vitamins A, D, and E; protein; and monounsaturated fats. These helpful substances might counteract the damage done by the cholesterol.

A Kansas State University study sheds more light on the egg puzzle. Professor Sung I. Koo and colleagues found that a compound in eggs called lecithin reduces the amount of cholesterol your body absorbs.

"This may be a reason why so many studies found no association between egg intake and blood cholesterol," Koo says. "Less absorption means less cholesterol introduced into the blood. We were able to determine experimentally that a substantial amount of egg cholesterol is not going into the bloodstream."

Part of the danger of eggs is that they go so well with bacon. People who eat a lot of eggs may also tend to eat an unhealthy diet including bacon, red meat, whole milk, and few fruits and vegetables. That's a bad idea if you're watching your cholesterol.

Just in case its message about eggs got scrambled somewhere along the way, the American Heart Association recently clarified that an egg a day is fine — as long as you keep your total cholesterol to 300 milligrams (mg) or less. Because an egg averages 213 mg of cholesterol, limit your dietary cholesterol from other sources.

Get creative with egg substitutes

While you're enjoying your egg-a-day allowance, don't forget to count the eggs in baked goods. Try these egg substitutes when baking to keep your cholesterol levels down.

- ▸ For each egg called for, mix together 1 1/2 tablespoons of water, 1 1/2 tablespoons of oil, and 1 teaspoon of baking powder.

- ▸ Stir 1 envelope of unflavored gelatin into 1 cup of boiling water. Store in your refrigerator and microwave the mixture when you want to use it. For each egg, substitute 3 tablespoons of the liquid.

- ▸ Use two egg whites for one whole egg in recipes or on your breakfast plate. Egg white is high in protein, riboflavin, and lysine, and it does almost everything whole eggs do — but without the tiniest hint of fat or cholesterol.

2 steps toward lower cholesterol

Is high cholesterol threatening your heart health? Bring it down one step at a time using one of the Step diets – eating plans developed by the National Institutes of Health.

While your body needs cholesterol to help make vitamin D, hormones, and even digestive juices, a little goes a long way. And most people have far more cholesterol than they need, especially the dangerous kind called low-density lipoprotein (LDL) cholesterol. Excess cholesterol travels to the walls of your arteries and causes fatty buildup, a condition called atherosclerosis. This significantly raises your risk of angina, stroke, and heart attacks.

That's where Step comes in. Endorsed by both the American Heart Association and the National Cholesterol Education Program (NCEP), the Step program guides you through simple diet changes proven to reduce your LDL cholesterol. Foods containing saturated fat and animal-based cholesterol can send your blood cholesterol skyrocketing. To rein it in, the Step diets encourage you to cut back on these foods and build a better balance of fibrous, nutrient-rich foods. The Step eating plan has two levels.

▶ Step I, a preventive diet for people who need to lower their cholesterol but don't yet suffer from heart disease

▶ Step II, for those at high risk for heart disease or who already have it

Generally, Step II is stricter than Step I, but both can help lower your cholesterol. The guidelines depend on how many calories you usually eat each day. As your calories change, so does the amount of fat you can eat. Some larger or very active people may eat up to 2,400 calories a day, while those who are petite or less active may only need around 1,500 calories.

The following quick comparison should give you an idea of your daily goals for fat, cholesterol, and calories under each program. Check the fat and cholesterol amounts on food nutrition labels to be sure you keep within your range.

	Step I	Step II
Saturated fat	no more than 8 to 10 percent of your daily calories	no more than 7 percent of your daily calories
Total fat	less than 30 percent of your daily calories	less than 30 percent of your daily calories
Cholesterol	less than 300 mg each day	less than 200 mg each day
Calories	a controlled amount to keep a healthy weight	a controlled amount to keep a healthy weight

Now here's a breakdown of the saturated and total fat you're allowed under each Step diet based on your daily calories. The fat here is measured in grams. To convert that to calories, just multiply the number of fat grams by 9 — since 1 gram of fat has 9 calories.

Saturated fat grams per day under Step plan

Calories	1,500	1,700	1,900	2,100	2,300
Step I at 9%	15	17	19	21	23
Step II at 6%	10	11	13	14	15

Total fat grams per day under Step plan

Steps I & II at 30%	50	57	63	70	77

Let's say you lower the amount of saturated fat calories you eat every day by just 1 percent. That lowers your body's LDL cholesterol by 1 percent. Every 1-percent drop in your cholesterol results in a 2-percent decrease in your risk of heart attack. Research shows the Step II diet could lower your cholesterol between 5 and 20 percent, while Step I may yield more modest results. Not bad for such a small change in diet. These guidelines on specific food groups will help you stay in step.

Harvest a healthier heart. Plant foods form the foundation of the Step diets, proving you can best lower your cholesterol by grazing on plants rather than gorging on meats. Grains and legumes are full of fiber and naturally lower your cholesterol. Fruits and vegetables deliver their own fiber punch alongside key vitamins, minerals, and antioxidants. Plus, most are amazingly low in sodium, calories, and saturated fat.

Get the deal on dairy. As an animal food, dairy products can be loaded with saturated fat. Make the switch to low-fat dairy, like skim or 1-percent milk, nonfat yogurt, and low-fat cheese and ice cream. You'll get crucial nutrients without the danger of excess fat. Some fats, like sphingolipids, are valuable for good health. In animal studies, these lipids lowered bad LDL cholesterol and raised good HDL cholesterol. They are found in dairy foods, including 1-percent low-fat milk, and eggs.

Pick lean meat. Red and processed meats are major sources of saturated fat. Buy the leanest cuts you can, and opt for fish and poultry. Even then, keep your portions small, less than 6 ounces a day. That's equal in size to about two decks of playing cards.

Give eggs a break. Egg yolks are high in saturated fat and cholesterol, although it's the fat, not the cholesterol, that does the most damage. Step I allows you to eat up to four egg yolks in a week. Step II is stricter, limiting you to two yolks each week. Remember, you probably get more eggs than you think – they're hidden in all kinds of baked goods. So skip the yolks altogether and cook with egg whites or an egg substitute, when possible.

Know your oils. Prepare foods with monounsaturated fatty oils, such as olive and canola, or with polyunsaturated oils, like safflower, corn, and soybean. These seem to help lower your cholesterol if you use them in small amounts. But don't overdo it – they still contribute to your total fat calories.

Discuss the Step program with your doctor, a registered dietitian, or a nutrition specialist. They can track your results, give you tips, and encourage you to stick with it. Get going – and take the first step toward lowering your cholesterol.

Diet defense

8 weeks to a healthier mind and body

Feel younger, healthier, and more energetic

There's no denying you are what you eat. And no matter how old you are, good nutrition is important. You need nutrients to build muscles and strengthen bones, as well as stay active all day long. What you eat even affects your risk for illnesses, like heart disease, cancer, and osteoporosis. In fact, proper nutrition can help you manage many symptoms you already have.

Your brain needs good food, too. A nutritionally balanced eating plan can keep you mentally young and protect you from memory loss, depression, Alzheimer's disease, and other mental disorders. It's clear eating right can help you stay independent and active, maintain a higher quality of life, and enjoy a longer one.

The *Complete Nutrition* eating plan you'll read about in this chapter puts you on that path, without guesswork or drastic diet changes. It's specifically designed to meet the nutritional needs of older adults and lower your risk for many serious illnesses. You'll gradually alter your eating habits one week – and one step – at a time. In just eight weeks, you should feel younger, healthier, and more energetic.

Best of all, the eating plan is super simple. You start with a healthy foundation based on plenty of water every day, then build in whole grains, fruits, and vegetables. Add in dairy, legumes, fish, nuts, seeds, and an occasional serving of meat. Finally, you'll learn how to go easy with sweets and snacks.

Start each week thinking about how that food group fits into your current eating habits. Then slowly make the recommended change – one change per week. You'll either eat more of – or cut back on – a certain kind of food. By week's end, your new eating habit will feel like second nature, and you'll be one step closer to a healthier, happier you.

This eight-week *Complete Nutrition* eating plan is designed to keep both your body and your brain fit. It's a recipe for longevity based on well-balanced, age-defying eating habits. The healthier your mind and body are, the likelier you are to live a long, full life – even to 100 and beyond.

However, food isn't the whole story. You also need to make healthy lifestyle choices, like exercising regularly, getting plenty of sleep, wearing a seat belt, and quitting smoking. Not surprisingly, nutritious eating habits give you an edge.

Week 1

Turn back the clock with water

Explorers searched for it, civilizations fought over it, and now corporations bottle and sell it for billions of dollars a year. With all the excitement over this natural resource, it only makes sense that water forms the foundation of your new eating plan.

In your first week on the *Complete Nutrition* eating plan, in addition to your regular menu, you'll start drinking more water and other healthy beverages. By the end of the week, you should be up and running on eight 8-ounce servings a day. Feeling like a fish? Read on to find out how fluids keep your body in tip-top condition, and what other food and drinks you can substitute for water.

Creative ways to drink more water

If you're tired of drinking plain ol' water, these beverages also supply water. One serving of water equals 8 ounces of:

- ▶ tea
- ▶ juice
- ▶ reduced-sodium soup
- ▶ coffee
- ▶ nonfat milk

Drink up and reap the rewards

You could survive nearly a month without food but only a few days without water. It's crucial for keeping your body cool during exercise — especially if you're outdoors — and you need it to replace the fluids you lose through sweat.

You can't beat its health benefits, either. Water carries the nutrients you eat to every cell in your body. It cushions joints, regulates body temperature, and lubricates your digestive tract. It's famous for soothing gout, arthritis, heartburn, and other uncomfortable digestive problems. It can even successfully ward off kidney stones, gallstones, and urinary tract infections.

This divine drink is also a dieter's dream. Water has no fat, sugar, or calories, but it's no empty-headed beverage, either. It can provide Grade A nutrition, mostly in the form of minerals. Your drinking water might contain fluoride, a mineral known for protecting teeth and bones, as well as magnesium, calcium, or iron. If your water comes to you through copper pipes, you're likely getting more of – you guessed it – copper.

Hard water for health

Rates of heart disease are much lower in areas where the water is "hard." The calcium and magnesium salts in most hard water help your heart maintain a good balance of electrolytes for trouble-free function. If you live in one of these areas, a chlorine-removing filter would be a better choice than bottled water. If not, a bottled water that is hard or contains minerals is better than one that is "soft." Avoid distilled water, which is free of minerals.

How much water should you drink?

You've probably heard the "8 x 8 rule" – drink eight 8-ounce glasses of water every day. New research suggests most people need about eight servings of water-containing drinks or food each day. So if the idea of guzzling eight glasses of water isn't appealing, try substituting an occasional 8 ounces of soup, tea, low-calorie juice, or nonfat milk.

Making these swaps every once in a while is all right, but don't leave out water entirely. Nothing beats water as the original thirst quencher. If you're over age 70, exercise vigorously, or have certain medical conditions such as kidney stones, you may actually need eight or more glasses of water every day. Check with your doctor if you have special medical needs.

Not drinking enough water is a much greater health risk for most people than drinking too much. But how can you tell how much fluid you need when requirements can vary? Here's a simple rule that most people can follow. Urine output increases when you drink too much water and decreases when you don't get enough. If you're not producing at least one quart of urine per 24 hours, you're probably not drinking enough. Not sure how to estimate your urine output? It's helpful to know your bladder can comfortably hold about one cup of urine before the urge to urinate and must be emptied when it contains two cups of urine. If you're producing two or more quarts each day, you're drinking more than enough fluids and possibly too much. Adjust your drinking habits accordingly.

Drinking too much water can dilute your electrolytes, a condition called water intoxication. Severe cases may be life threatening. In at least one case, a 45-year-old woman developed water intoxication by drinking large quantities of water to suppress her appetite. Even during heavy exertion in high heat, the U.S. Army has warned its members against drinking more than six 8-ounce glasses of water in an hour or more than 48 8-ounce glasses in 12 hours.

Drinking too much water is a real concern but not as likely as dehydration, a dangerous condition that can lead to seizures, coma, or even death. Ignoring these warning signs could be deadly.

- ▸ dry lips and mouth
- ▸ dizziness or headaches
- ▸ forgetfulness, confusion
- ▸ rapid breathing
- ▸ increased heart rate
- ▸ dark urine, constipation
- ▸ weakness, lack of energy

Not all waters are created equal

No water is naturally pure, no matter its source. It all picks up pollutants, like bacteria and chemicals. The main differences between bottled and tap water are how each is cleaned and how they taste.

Public drinking water is generally purified with chlorine, which can leave a flavor or odor behind. Free chlorine is a very harmful free radical. The small chlorine residual in tap water may have an insidious adverse effect on health. Bottled water is often filtered, or treated with ultraviolet light or with some form of oxygen. These methods sometimes make bottled water taste "cleaner" than chlorinated tap water.

You need plenty of water for good health and tap water is better than no water. However, if you have a choice, bottled water or a filter that removes chlorine at your water tap is better.

The federal government regulates both bottled and public water for safety. The Environmental Protection Agency (EPA) tests public drinking water, while the Food and Drug Administration (FDA) sets standards for bottled water. If you reuse water bottles, wash them out with hot, soapy water to keep bacteria from building up.

Week 2

Guard against health problems with grains

Grains are an energy powerhouse, feeding your body like dry logs on a fire. In fact, most of your daily fuel should come from this food group. Grains, especially whole-grain foods, keep you fit on the outside by giving you energy to walk or swim, garden or golf.

In addition, they keep you fit on the inside by toning your digestive tract. Besides that, nutrients in grains are known to ward off heart disease, strokes, cancer, constipation, and mental illness.

Beginning in week two of your *Complete Nutrition* eating plan, you'll continue drinking eight glasses of water a day and eating your normal menu. In addition, you'll focus on getting at least six servings of grains a day — preferably whole grains. Servings are often smaller than you think, so they add up fast.

For instance, one grain serving equals just half a medium bagel, one slice of bread, a cup of dry cereal, or half a cup of cooked cereal, pasta, or rice.

Begin making grains a standard part of every meal and snack, and you'll soon meet the challenge of your second week. Check out these not-to-be-missed tips on choosing the best grains for good health.

Put your flour to the test

The less refined the flour, the more nutrients it contains. Run your flour through a sifter. If most won't pass through, it's coarse and unprocessed enough to provide healthy benefits.

Maximize benefits with whole grains

Starch, sugar, and fiber — known collectively as carbohydrates — give grains their get-up-and-go. Without carbs, you wouldn't have the energy to climb out of bed. Carbs come almost exclusively from plant foods, including grains, fruits, and vegetables. Chances are you get many of your carbs from breads, pasta, cereals, and other grains. But buyer beware — not all carbohydrates are equal.

Dr. Walter C. Willett, professor of nutrition and medicine at Harvard University and author of *Eat, Drink, and Be Healthy*, warns that the kind of carbs you get from highly processed grains — like white bread and refined flour — may actually do more harm than good. That's partly because your body digests these refined carbs with lightning speed. Your blood sugar and insulin levels shoot through the roof and quickly plummet back to earth, leaving you hungry again.

177

According to Willett, the long-term results of a diet based on refined grains are higher triglycerides, lower HDL (good) cholesterol, and an increased risk for heart disease, diabetes, and weight gain.

Whole-grain foods, on the other hand, undergo much less processing than refined grains, so they keep more of their original nutrients. The carbs in whole grains also digest more slowly, stabilizing your insulin and blood sugar and giving you longer-lasting energy. Add it up, and whole grains may lower your risk for heart disease, digestive cancers, diabetes, and diverticulosis.

About half of your day's energy, as measured in calories, should come from carbohydrates. Grains are a great source, but choose wisely. Go with whole-wheat pastas, breads, and flour; brown rice; whole or steel-cut oats; and other healthy whole grains whenever possible. You may discover new foods, appreciate new tastes, and perhaps live longer in the process.

Why you need more fiber

Want to stay off prescription drugs? Grains pack an especially potent punch of fiber, a kind of carbohydrate famous for its health benefits. Experts believe fiber helps lower cholesterol, as well as prevent diverticulosis, constipation, weight gain, diabetes, and possibly even colon cancer. Fibrous foods also fill you up, so you tend to eat less.

Fiber comes in two forms – soluble and insoluble. Soluble fiber dissolves in water, whereas insoluble doesn't. Each plays a crucial role in long-term health by providing specific benefits. You'll find soluble fiber in dried beans and peas, oats, barley, flaxseed, and many fruits and vegetables. This kind of fiber turns soft in your body, slowing things down in your stomach and small intestine. This gives your body a better opportunity to whisk away harmful cholesterol and absorb carbohydrates more slowly, helping to control your blood sugar.

Your body can't break down insoluble fiber so the bulk of it passes through your digestive system, giving it a healthy workout. This keeps your bowels moving smoothly and tones your digestive muscles, guarding against constipation and diverticulosis. It may protect against colon cancer, too. Look for insoluble fiber in whole-wheat foods, bran, and fruits and vegetables with tough, chewy textures.

Most experts believe older adults don't eat enough fiber-rich foods. The Institute of Medicine recommends men over age 50 get at least 30 grams of fiber each day, and women the same age no less than 21 grams a day. Get six servings of grains every day to meet this goal. For the biggest boost, choose high-fiber whole grains instead of refined ones that are low in fiber.

Whole grains are a gold mine of many other nutrients, too — protein, zinc, magnesium, and manganese. Just remember to eat a variety of grains for a healthy heart.

5 ways to harvest more benefits

- Work grains gradually into your diet, especially if you eat very few now. This allows your body time to adjust to the extra fiber and nutrients.

- Look for foods with these whole grains first in their ingredient list: whole oats, whole wheat, whole rye, whole grain corn, oatmeal, brown rice, cracked wheat or bulgur, pearl barley, or graham flour. Beware of imposters. "Wheat flour," "enriched flour," and "degerminated corn meal" sound fancy, but they aren't whole grains.

- Pick brown rice over white. It's less refined and has triple the fiber of white rice.

- Read food labels to find a cereal that contains at least 5 grams of fiber per serving.

- Drink plenty of fluids as you eat more fiber to help your body digest it. Try to get your recommended eight servings of water or a good substitute.

Dangerous dosage turns good vitamin bad

Folate has a big assignment. It has a hand in building every cell in your body, especially red blood cells. It may lower your risk for heart disease, stroke, and certain kinds of cancer. However, according to recent studies, taking large amounts of folate as supplements may be a mixed blessing — a possible reduction in strokes but potential exacerbation of the growth of undetected cancer cells hiding in the body and ultimate increases in rates of cancer.

This multi-talented vitamin also helps keep your wits sharp and protects you from depression and other forms of "the blues." Both women and men over the age of 50 need about 400 micrograms (mcg) of folate daily. Manufacturers "enrich" many grain products by adding back some of the nutrients lost during processing. Enriched flour, pasta, bread, and cereal have added folate, as well as iron and the other B vitamins — thiamin, riboflavin, and niacin.

A single slice of bread won't give you enough folate for a day. Eat a variety of grain products, like fortified cereal, plus plenty of legumes and dark, leafy green vegetables to stay on track.

Antacids and aspirin products can interfere with how your body uses folate. Taking these medications occasionally shouldn't cause a problem, but if you use them often, talk to your doctor about a vitamin supplement. If you smoke or take estrogen, you may need to supplement, too.

Easy ways to eat more grains

▸ Try different grain products like whole grain muffins, rice, and pitas or more exotic grains, such as bulgur, quinoa, and kasha.

▸ Make hot or cold whole-grain cereal a regular part of your mornings.

▸ Top off tasty casseroles, soups, yogurt, or ice cream with a nutritious serving of cereal. Use it to bread fish before baking or sprinkle it on salad for a satisfying crunch.

▸ Throw cooked barley, brown rice, or whole-wheat pasta in with other foods like vegetables or soups.

Balance blood sugar with chromium

Without chromium, an important trace mineral, balancing your blood sugar can be a high-wire act. Chromium teams up with insulin to turn the sugars you eat into energy. While chromium won't cure diabetes, eating too little of this mineral can worsen the disease. What's more, research shows people who have diabetes are more likely to develop heart disease than people who don't have diabetes.

Men over the age of 50 should try to get 30 mcg of chromium a day, while women the same age need at least 20 mcg daily. Whole-grain foods are hands down the best source of chromium.

Just 2 ounces of shredded wheat cereal typically gives you 65 mcg of chromium — well over your daily goal. Nuts, cheese, eggs, and fish are also good sources of this mineral.

Vital mineral for heart health

Although your body needs only small amounts of selenium, it's vital for heart health. This powerful antioxidant helps keep your heart pumping oxygen-rich blood to every part of your body. It does this by helping to form prostaglandins, hormone-like fatty acids that can help lower blood pressure and prevent blood clots. Rates of heart disease are much lower when selenium is plentiful in foods and the water supply, but studies of taking selenium as a supplement have failed to show any benefit.

It also neutralizes free radicals, unstable molecules that damage cells through a process called oxidation. If left unchecked, free radicals would oxidize all your LDL cholesterol, making it even more damaging to your arteries. The more your arteries are damaged, the more plaque builds up on them and the narrower they become.

Your heart must work harder and your chance of developing life-threatening blood clots is greater. But antioxidants, like selenium, keep this from happening. Many studies have shown that people who eat foods rich in antioxidants have a lower risk of heart disease.

And there's more. Look to selenium if you want to feel young for as long as you live. This anti-aging mineral plays a major role in boosting your immune system and making thyroid hormones. It may even protect you against some kinds of cancer.

Men and women over age 50 should aim for 55 mcg of selenium each day. Plants, such as grains, absorb this mineral from the soil they are grown in. Six servings of whole grains should provide you with all the selenium you need for the day.

As you progress through the *Complete Nutrition* eating plan, you'll add other foods rich in selenium to your diet — like vegetables and lean meats.

Week 3

Age gracefully with fruits and veggies

It's week three of your *Complete Nutrition* eating plan and you should be used to getting plenty of water and whole grains every day. But you're not through, yet. Now, you need to add more fruits and vegetables.

Some foods do more than give you energy — they actually help you stay young. Fruits and vegetables are long-life foods, packed with nutrients to help slow down the aging process and prevent disease.

Vitamins and minerals are keys to healthy aging, and the foods in this group are loaded with both. Even better, most are low in fat, cholesterol-free, and naturally filling. Unfortunately, the U.S. Department of Agriculture found most people don't eat enough fruits and vegetables to enjoy the amazing benefits.

Research shows you could drop your blood pressure and cholesterol, as well as lower your risk for heart disease and cancer just by eating plenty of fruits and vegetables. Getting more home-grown nutrition from these foods is a delicious way to keep your heart healthy, and it's unbelievably easy.

During the third week of your *Complete Nutrition* eating plan, begin building in a total of six servings of veggies and fruits every day. One serving equals a half cup berries; one cup raw, leafy vegetables; a half cup cooked or raw vegetables; one-quarter cup dried fruit; or three-quarters cup juice.

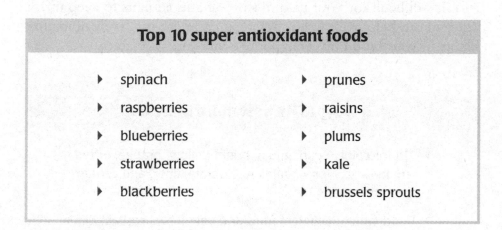

Top 10 super antioxidant foods

▶ spinach	▶ prunes
▶ raspberries	▶ raisins
▶ blueberries	▶ plums
▶ strawberries	▶ kale
▶ blackberries	▶ brussels sprouts

Put the brakes on free radicals

When you cut open an apple, oxygen in the air reacts with it, creating unstable compounds called free radicals. These compounds damage the apple, turning it brown.

The same thing happens in your body. You breathe in oxygen, and your body processes it, creating free radicals at the same time. These unstable molecules travel through your body looking for electrons they can steal from healthy cells in order to become stable. When they succeed, they leave the cell irreversibly damaged. This is called oxidation.

Of course, you don't necessarily see the damage as you do with the apple. It happens at a much slower pace, but the harm free radicals cause increases over time. Researchers have linked free radical damage to over 200 diseases, including heart disease, cataracts, diabetes, and some cancers.

Antioxidants are a family of nutrients that can put the brakes on free radicals. This special group includes vitamins A, C, and E. The minerals selenium, copper, zinc, and manganese, and some nutrients called phytochemicals also act as antioxidants. They fight oxidation by combining with free radicals to keep them stable and harmless. Oxidation is probably going on in your body right now.

In addition, cigarette smoke, pollution, radiation, stress, excessive sun exposure, and other factors can increase your level of free radicals. It's difficult for your natural store of antioxidants to keep up, but you can help. Research proves you can raise the levels of antioxidants in your blood by eating more fruits and vegetables.

5 ways to harvest more benefits

▶ Go for color — dark green, bright yellow, orange, or red are best bets for vitamins A, C, folate, fiber, and certain phytochemicals.

▶ Eat a variety. Different fruits and vegetables contain different nutrients, and you need them all to fortify your body.

▶ Cook vegetables lightly to preserve the important phytochemicals inside them.

▶ Try to eat fruits and veggies whole or sliced instead of always drinking them as juices. Liquids often lack the fiber in the original food.

▶ Don't let mouth or tooth problems stand in your way of good health. Grate, chop, or purée crunchy vegetables if you have a hard time chewing them.

Arm yourself with vitamin C

In your fight for good health, vitamin C may be your greatest weapon. Vitamin C is a building block of collagen, the tissue that holds your bones, muscles, and joints together, and it's well-known for strengthening your immune system to help fight colds, heal wounds, and prevent infections. It's a powerful antioxidant, too, so when you eat vitamin C-rich foods you're fending off free radical damage.

A woman over age 50 needs about 75 milligrams (mg) of vitamin C each day. Men the same age need more — 90 mg a day. These are the official recommendations. However, many studies indicate the optimal amount of daily vitamin C probably is more, perhaps three or four times higher. Citrus fruits, like oranges and grapefruit, are chock-full of vitamin C, but colorful fruits — strawberries, kiwis, tomatoes, and cantaloupe — aren't far behind. Broccoli, peppers, potatoes, and leafy greens, like romaine lettuce and cabbage, carry loads of vitamin C. Six servings of fruits and vegetables every day should serve you well. Dish out a variety for a delicious, healthy dose of vitamin C.

Defend your heart with phytochemicals

Plants contain natural chemicals, called phytochemicals or phytonutrients, that protect them from disease, drought, too much sun, and even bugs. Fortunately, these built-in defenders can help people, too. When you eat colorful plant foods, you wind up eating hundreds of phytochemicals, as well.

Many of these special nutrients seem to boost your immune system and guard against deadly illnesses, like heart disease, stroke, and cancer. Some even act as antioxidants. Two, in particular, are becoming famous for their disease-fighting power.

▶ Beta carotene is just one of over 600 dyes found in plants. That makes it easy to spot a food rich in this nutrient — look for bright orange, red, or green fruits and vegetables. As an antioxidant, beta carotene has a knack for preventing heart disease, cancer, memory loss, and rheumatoid arthritis. It even helps save your eyesight as you age. Carrots, for one, are crammed with beta carotene, as are other orange vegetables, like sweet potatoes, and delicious fruits, such as mangoes, cantaloupe, and

185

apricots. If you prefer greens, dig into the dark, leafy variety, especially spinach and collard greens.

▸ Lycopene, which gives fruits their red hue, could also give you a long lease on life. Research shows it may protect against prostate, stomach, and esophageal cancers. In addition, it helps preserve your eyesight. Watermelon, papaya, pink grapefruit, tomato products, and other pink or red fruits are full of this famous phytochemical.

Different phytochemicals come from different plants. For instance, oranges alone have over 170 different kinds. Cruciferous vegetables, such as beets, kale, cabbage, and broccoli, are also full of an assortment of antioxidant phytochemicals. Your best bet for all-round health is to make variety part of your daily menu.

Easy ways to eat more fruits and veggies

▸ Add an extra serving at each meal during week three until you reach your total of six a day.

▸ Slice up strawberries, peaches, or bananas on hot or cold cereal, or stir them into plain, low-fat yogurt.

▸ Leave meat out of one meal at least twice a week and add more vegetables instead.

▸ Toss extra fruits and vegetables into salads, soups, or casseroles.

▸ Don't settle for just meat and bread — dress sandwiches up with lettuce, tomato, cucumbers, sliced carrots, and green or red pepper.

▸ Try fruit as a sweet end to your meals instead of high-calorie, high-fat desserts.

▸ Keep a bag of dried fruits or fresh, sliced veggies at hand for snacking throughout the day.

Color your world healthy with vitamin A

Also called retinol, this antioxidant vitamin's job is to keep your cornea healthy, guarding your eyesight, particularly your night vision. It also protects your skin, lungs, and bladder from infections and boosts your immune system so you're better able to fight off illnesses.

Women over the age of 50 need about 700 micrograms (mcg) of vitamin A each day, and men the same age about 900 mcg. Only animal foods, such as milk, liver, and eggs, provide vitamin A. Because your body turns the phytochemical beta carotene into vitamin A, snacking like a rabbit is another great way to get more of this important vitamin. Look for beta carotene in bright orange and dark green vegetables and fruits.

Be careful. Taking too much vitamin A can be very dangerous. This is why it's better to get vitamin A from eating foods containing carotenes, which are converted into vitamin A only as needed by the body.

Keep your body moving with potassium

As you hike up that hill, perhaps you can feel your thigh muscles tighten and your heart beat just a little harder. That's all thanks to potassium. This mineral helps regulate your heartbeat, keeps your muscles and nerves working properly, and controls your blood pressure. What that means is you are able to walk, bike, garden, play tennis, and participate in just about any form of exercise you choose.

Fruits and vegetables pack in the potassium, but you can also get it from fish, legumes, and dairy products. That's good news since a healthy body needs lots of this mineral. Most men and women over 50 years old should aim for around 4,700 milligrams (mg) of potassium in their diets each day. People who take a potassium-sparing diuretic or have certain kidney or other health problems should check with their doctors because this amount of potassium may be too much. Potassium overdose can actually cause a heart attack in people who have taken large amounts of potassium supplements. That's why it's good to get most of your potassium from your daily diet.

A big number like that may sound daunting, but you'd be surprised how fast potassium adds up when you eat a variety of foods. One medium banana, for instance, provides 450 mg. By the end of week three, fit six servings of fruits and vegetables into your daily menu, and you should never come up short.

Fresh, canned, or frozen?

Food gurus often disdain frozen or canned fruits and vegetables. Their motto — fresh is best. Fresh, however, is a relative term. Most produce has a short shelf life. After they sit in your refrigerator or in your pantry for about three days, fresh foods start to lose their nutrients.

Truth is, frozen and canned veggies and fruits generally have the same nutritional value as their fresh relatives. If you can or flash freeze produce right off the vine, you lock in vitamins and minerals. The biggest drawbacks to processed foods are the added sodium and sugar. Check the Nutrition Facts label and find foods without these extras.

Many experts recommend you buy enough fresh food to last you about three days. Then, switch to canned or frozen until you're able to stock up again on produce.

Keep breaks at bay with vitamin K

Blood that clots and bones that don't break — you may take them for granted. But without vitamin K, chances are you wouldn't have either. This nutrient makes specific proteins that cause your blood to form clots and works hard alongside vitamin D to strengthen your bones.

In fact, a Harvard Medical School study found eating vegetables high in vitamin K could reduce your risk for hip fractures. People who eat a variety of veggies on a regular basis are usually OK on vitamin K. So if you fell off the turnip truck, climb back on. Green leafy vegetables, such as spinach and broccoli, are the kings of vitamin K, as are lettuce, cauliflower, and cabbage.

A word of caution – check with your doctor before eating foods high in vitamin K if you take blood-thinning drugs, like warfarin (Coumadin). Vitamin K will interfere with the action of these drugs.

The fruits and veggies group delivers nonstop nutrition, including superstars you already know about – carbohydrates, fiber, folate, and selenium, as well as those you'll see later in this chapter, such as vitamin B6 and the minerals magnesium, zinc, and calcium.

Toss together a diet teeming with different vegetables and fruits, and you have a remarkable recipe for good health. Dress your plate in these powerful plant foods, and lift your fork to a long, happy life.

Week 4

Stay stronger, longer with dairy

By the fourth week of your *Complete Nutrition* eating plan, you've built a healthy daily menu based on plenty of water, grains, fruits, and vegetables. Now, it's time to think about how much dairy you get every day. You don't have to be young to benefit from this food group. It's the basis of strong bones and youthful activity at any age.

The bad news is one in three white men and women will break a hip by age 90. Blacks and Hispanics have only a slightly smaller risk. While a broken bone is certainly disabling, the worst news is one out of four people die from complications within six months of breaking a hip.

A dairy-filled eating plan and regular exercise could extend not only your independence but also your life. The nutrients in these foods shore up weakening bones, shielding you from crippling diseases, like osteoporosis.

Write your own prescription for bone health and an active lifestyle by making sure you get three servings of dairy every day beginning in week four of your *Complete Nutrition* eating plan. One dairy serving equals an 8-ounce glass of milk, 2 ounces of hard cheese, or 8 ounces of yogurt.

How much fat is in fat-free milk?

The next time you're shopping for milk, consider these facts. Nonfat or skim milk has about .4 grams of fat in an 8-ounce glass and 1 percent or low-fat milk has about 2.4 grams of fat. Whole milk has a whopping 9 grams of fat in an 8-ounce glass. Compared to whole milk:

▶ Reduced-fat milk has 38 percent less fat.

▶ Low-fat milk has 63 percent less fat.

▶ Fat-free milk has 93 percent less fat. (Yes, Virginia, there is fat in fat-free milk.)

The small amount of fat remaining in fat-free milk is mostly sphingolipid, named after the dual-natured sphinx. Sphingolipids are mainly good fats that can help your heart, unlike the saturated butterfat that is the main fat in whole milk.

Count on calcium's many benefits

Bones are like a bank — your body uses them to store about 99 percent of its calcium. But your body also withdraws this mineral as it's needed. And it's needed for many functions — regulating blood pressure, sending nerve impulses, contracting muscles, and clotting your blood, to name a few. The trouble starts when you withdraw more calcium than you deposit. Just like a bank account, you could end up in the red — with fragile bones and osteoporosis.

The solution is to get enough calcium in your diet to replace what you borrow from your bones every day. That's why it's never too late for more calcium. Both men and women over the age of 50 should get at least 1,200 milligrams (mg) daily. Many experts believe postmenopausal women – not taking estrogen – need even more calcium. Their recommendation for this group is 1,500 mg a day. This is a snap if you follow the three-a-day dairy recommendation. However, your body won't be able to absorb the calcium it needs from your intestines if you don't have a liberal amount of vitamin D in your system. Read more information about the optimal amounts of vitamin D in this chapter.

Dairy foods, like milk, yogurt, and cheese, are some of the best natural sources of calcium. An 8-ounce container of nonfat plain yogurt starts you off with 450 mg of calcium. Add a cup of low-fat milk for another 300 mg, and an ounce of cheddar or part-skim mozzarella cheese for about 200 more milligrams.

Some cold breakfast cereals are loaded with up to 1,000 mg of calcium per serving, while leafy green vegetables, fortified juices, and fish with small, edible bones, such as sardines or salmon, can round out your intake of this essential nutrient. Your doctor may also suggest a calcium supplement, but don't rely on that alone to build your bones. Instead, make it part of a healthy, dairy-filled diet.

4 ways to reap more benefits

▸ Read the Nutrition Facts label on dairy and other foods, and buy those with the fewest grams of saturated fat.

▸ Realize that not all dairy foods offer the same nutrients. Cottage cheese and frozen yogurt treats have half the calcium of milk. Butter, cream, and cream cheese are mostly fat with very little calcium.

▸ Look for lactose-free dairy products if you have trouble digesting regular dairy. Or buy milk with lactase enzyme added to it.

▸ Consider drinking soy milk with added calcium if you can't drink milk. Or try yogurt – it digests more easily.

Strengthen your body with phosphorus

This mineral forms the second piece of the strong-bone puzzle. It binds to calcium in your teeth and bones, adding extra might to these hard body parts. It's essential to every cell in your body, not just your bones, for its ability to carry, store, and release the energy you get from food. Dairy products provide plenty of phosphorus. You should have no trouble getting 700 mg a day of this mineral, the recommendation for people over age 50.

Warning – too much phosphorus in your diet can draw calcium out of your bones, weakening them. You'll find high amounts of phosphoric acid, a form of phosphorus, in cola drinks. Therefore, it's good to avoid them.

Meat, poultry, eggs, fish, nuts, and legumes also help satisfy your phosphorus requirements – more proof that a diverse diet can help you meet your nutritional needs naturally.

Defend your heart with vitamin D

Here's some sunny news for your heart – boosting your levels of vitamin D may lower your risk of heart-related death. A recent Austrian study found that people with the lowest blood levels of vitamin D were more than twice as likely to die from heart-related causes than those with the highest levels. Low vitamin D levels also led to more inflammation, oxidative stress, and cell adhesion – all factors that contribute to heart disease.

Vitamin D may also help keep your blood pressure in check. New Zealand researchers found that people with higher blood levels of vitamin D had lower blood pressure.

Your body produces vitamin D when exposed to sunshine, so spending more time in the sun can help. You can also get vitamin D from fortified foods, like milk and cereal, and supplements.

But most nutritional authorities think you need much more vitamin D than you get from most supplements and additions to foods. This is especially true if you don't get much direct exposure to sunshine when the sun is high on the horizon. Most adults should get 1,000 to 2,000 international units (IU) per day for optimal health in the absence of enough sun exposure, according to the Linus Pauling Institute.

Vitamin D products of sufficient strength are now available. Spring Valley's vitamin D3 is available in 1,000 IU strength. You can find it at your local discount store, drugstore, or online at *www.springvalleyherbs.com*. Nutraceutical Sciences Institute (NSI) sells vitamin D3 in 1,000 and 2,000 IU capsules. You can order them from 800-776-2887 or online at *www.gonsi.com*.

Be careful — too much vitamin D from supplements can be toxic. Your doctor can order a blood test to make sure you are taking a safe amount.

Depend on vitamin D for healthy bones

Vitamin D is vital for an active lifestyle because it helps your body absorb and use both calcium and phosphorus. According to the American Dietetic Association, your vitamin D intake is a big factor in your muscle strength, fracture risk, and bone health.

Steer clear of saturated fat

Fat may be the only downside to dairy foods. Most whole dairy foods are high in fat, particularly saturated fat — the kind best known for raising your cholesterol and your risk for heart disease, diabetes, and cancer. Yet, you still need three servings of dairy a day.

Compromise by choosing your dairy carefully. Low-fat and nonfat or fat-free milk, cheese, and yogurt contain the same nutrients as their regular versions but with much less saturated fat. They're excellent alternatives for getting your fill of calcium, phosphorus, and vitamin D without sacrificing your overall health.

Dairy products deliver other nutrition as well, making them all the more meaningful to a healthy eating plan. So while you're savoring yogurt or guzzling milk, appreciate the fact you're putting protein, potassium, and vitamins like A and B12 in your body, too.

7 easy ways to eat more dairy foods

▶ Have a glass of milk with a meal in place of soda, sweetened tea, coffee, or alcohol.

▶ Flavor your coffee and tea with milk instead of instant or non-dairy creamers. And use milk rather than water to make hot cereals, cocoa, and soups.

▶ Along with your milk, stir plain yogurt into your morning cereal.

▶ Sprinkle cheese on salads, soups, casseroles, or hot pastas.

▶ Add a dash of dry milk powder along with your regular milk in hot foods and recipes.

▶ Replace milk with low-fat versions of yogurt, buttermilk, cheese, or kefir, a yogurt-based drink. Or occasionally substitute 8 ounces of calcium-fortified juice for 8 ounces of milk.

▶ Pair up sliced cheese with crackers or fruit for a wholesome dairy-rich treat.

Week 5

Zap high cholesterol with legumes

In the story of Jack and the beanstalk, Jack sold his family's last cow for three legendary legumes. This boy knew the value of beans. You, on the other hand, don't have to sacrifice your family's source of income to share in the wealth of legumes. For pennies a day, you can make them part of your healthy diet.

Legumes are plants that develop their seeds inside pods. Think about how many foods fit that description, and you'll understand the variety you have to choose from. Beans, peas, lentils, peanuts, and soybeans all offer flavorful, unbeatable nutrition.

Most legumes are low in saturated fat but high in carbohydrates and healthy fiber — as well as top-notch nutrients, like protein, magnesium, and the B vitamin biotin.

Legumes have obvious health benefits, like keeping you regular, but there are subtle ones, too. They help control your cholesterol and blood sugar and cut your risk for heart disease and colon cancer. As if that's not enough — they are a waist-watcher's dream, satisfying your hunger longer than most other foods.

During week five of the *Complete Nutrition* eating plan, add one serving of legumes — a half cup of tofu, a half cup of beans, or two tablespoons of natural peanut butter — a day to your healthy menu. With so many varieties of beans and ways to prepare them, that should be easy.

4 easy ways to eat more legumes

▸ Make legumes, not meat, the center of a meal several times a week.

▸ Substitute legumes for a serving of meat or vegetables. Half a cup of cooked beans equals one vegetable serving, while a whole cup equals one meat serving.

▸ Add cooked beans, peas, or lentils to salads for fresh flavor and extra texture.

▸ Serve canned, frozen, or fresh beans rather than the dried ones when you're short on time.

Pack a powerful punch with protein

Like carbohydrates, protein packs lots of energy, but it's also essential to many body processes, like building muscles, bones, tendons, and ligaments. Proper protein can even give a healthy glow to your skin and hair.

There are several kinds of protein, some from plants like legumes, and others found in animal foods, like meat and dairy products. Beans alone don't provide all the different proteins, but they give you a strong start. Then you can round out your nutrition by eating foods such as grains, vegetables, fish, dairy, seeds, and nuts – other good sources of protein – throughout the day.

Based on a 2,000-calorie-a-day diet, men over 50 years old should get 56 grams of protein a day, while women the same age need a little less, about 46 grams.

5 ways to harvest more benefits

▸ Cut back on gas from dry beans by pouring out the water you soak them in and cooking them in fresh water. The beans, not the water, hold most of the nutrients.

▸ Soak raw beans at least five hours and boil them for a minimum of 10 minutes. Certain kinds of legumes – such as red kidney beans – are poisonous raw.

▸ Wait to add salt or acidic foods, like tomatoes and vinegar, to beans at the last minute. They keep beans from softening and can slow down cooking time.

▸ Eat tomatoes, lettuce, citrus fruits, or other foods high in vitamin C with legumes. The vitamin C helps your body absorb the iron from legumes.

▸ Add one-fourth teaspoon of cooking oil to a pot of beans to keep them from foaming over as they cook.

Muscle up with magnesium

This mineral steadies your heartbeat and helps your muscles contract and relax. It also prevents charley horses, those painful muscle cramps that can put a quick end to physical activity.

Experts recommend women over age 50 get 320 milligrams (mg) of this mineral each day and men get 420 mg. You'll fill your magnesium bill easily by following the *Complete Nutrition* eating plan since most beans are sensational sources.

One cup of boiled soybeans yields almost 150 mg. A cup of cooked navy beans provides another 100 mg. Other plant foods, such as grains, spinach, and nuts, also contribute this magnificent mineral.

When you wash and peel foods, however, you lose much of their natural magnesium. When you can, choose mostly whole, unprocessed foods. Some laxatives and antacids contain added magnesium. Taking too many regularly can overload your system. Read labels and use over-the-counter medications only as directed.

Maximize energy with biotin

This B vitamin helps your body transform the protein, carbohydrates, and fats you eat into energy for your daily routine, whether working in the garden or chasing grandchildren. It also helps your body use other B vitamins.

Your body doesn't need much biotin to run smoothly. Women and men 50 years or older require just 30 micrograms (mcg) a day from foods like legumes, cereal, or cauliflower. Peanuts are particularly rich in biotin — just 3 ounces of peanut butter fills the bill for this B vitamin.

These are just a few of the big-name nutrients legumes provide. Foods in this family also contain potassium, phosphorus, folate, and thiamin. Add the minerals — calcium, iron, zinc, and boron — and you have a nutritional powerhouse on your plate. Make a point to eat a serving of legumes every day during week five.

Week 6

'Go fish' for heart health

It's not just a leisurely pastime or even a card game. Fishing is now first aid for your heart. Whether you hook them at the lake or at the supermarket, eating fish at least twice a week could sink your risk for heart disease and stroke.

And thanks to healthy fats that prevent blood clots and improve your circulation, you could slash your stroke risk in half. In fact, the American Heart Association prescribes fish as a first line of treatment for warding off high blood pressure and heart attacks.

If that's not enough, you'll also do your joints a favor – studies show fishy diets may help tame arthritis. There's evidence, too, that fish could combat diabetes, cataracts, Alzheimer's disease, depression, and a host of other age-related illnesses.

Baked or broiled, fish is a nutritional winner. It's low in artery-clogging saturated fats, cholesterol, and calories and loaded with amazing unsaturated fats, vitamins, and minerals.

Start week six of your *Complete Nutrition* eating plan by serving fish at least twice a week. One fish serving equals a cooked filet about the size of a deck of cards. Keep in mind, fish cooks down, so start with a 4-ounce raw filet to end up with 3 ounces of cooked fish.

---

4 easy ways to eat more fish

▶ Grill or roast fish kebabs using firm, fatty fish, like salmon or tuna.

▶ Dress poached fish with fresh herbs and wine or reduced-sodium bouillon.

▶ Bake fish on a bed of thinly sliced vegetables and olive oil. Top each serving with fresh basil and mushrooms.

▶ Add cooked fish to a leafy green salad for a light, nutritious meal.

Perk up your heart with polyunsaturated fats

Some types of fats, such as saturated fats and trans fats – harmful fats you'll learn more about in week eight – can raise your cholesterol. But others, known as unsaturated fats, actually seem to lower your cholesterol.

Omega-3 fatty acids are polyunsaturated fatty acids (PUFAs) found mainly in fish. Experts with the American Heart Association believe the omega-3 in fish can have a huge impact on your heart. Eaten regularly, these super fats:

▸ rein in high blood pressure.

▸ reduce triglyceride levels.

▸ lower your chances for dangerous blood clots.

▸ slow down plaque build-up in your arteries.

▸ decrease your risk of arrhythmia, an irregular heartbeat, and sudden death.

But the fats in fish don't stop there. Some experts believe a fish-filled diet could keep your mind sharp as you age. The protective effects of omega-3 fatty acids kick in quickly. Even if you haven't eaten fish all your life, you could start now and still reap the benefits just by eating fatty fish twice a week.

People who already have heart disease should talk to their doctor about healthy diet changes, like adding more fish to help get their illness under control.

As you build your heart-healthy menu, remember that fried fish from restaurants, fast-food establishments, and your grocer's freezer don't count. In fact, skip these altogether. Fish prepared this way contains little omega-3 but lots of dangerous trans fats.

Fish may be the richest source of omega-3 fatty acids, but it's not the only one. Go ahead and up your intake by broiling or baking your fish with omega-3-rich canola or soybean oil, and adding English walnuts or ground flaxseed to your meals.

Iron out weakness and fatigue

It's often associated with strength, and no wonder. Iron is your body's pack horse. It helps make hemoglobin, a substance in red blood cells. Hemoglobin carries oxygen from your lungs to every cell in your body.

If you're low in this mineral, you'll feel too tired to climb out of bed and too weak to face the day. An iron deficiency is easy to fix since once you're over age 50 you only need about 8 mg a day.

Red meat has plenty of iron but there is far less in fish and poultry. Your body easily absorbs the form of iron found in these foods. Legumes and some vegetables, however, provide a different form — the type your body has more difficulty absorbing.

Look to legumes and enriched grains to give you iron on the days you don't eat fish. Meats generally are rich sources, too. Later in this chapter, you'll read important information about how to make meat a healthy part of your eating plan.

Think twice before taking iron supplements

Taking iron supplements may not be good for you, unless you are a woman who has irregular monthly bleeding. A recent study looked to see if there was a cardiovascular benefit from lowering the body's amount of iron by donating blood. The results were unexpected — no benefit for heart disease but a dramatic reduction in the rate of cancer in those who gave blood. Apparently, lots of iron, especially the heme iron found in red meat, may be more helpful for cancer cells than normal cells.

7 ways to reap more benefits

▶ Reel in Atlantic salmon, herring, mackerel, sardines, or rainbow trout for the most omega-3 fatty acids. Pacific oysters are a terrific source, as well.

▶ Serve fish with a side of beans to boost your iron. The iron in animal foods helps your body absorb the iron from plant foods, like legumes.

▶ Eat a variety of fish to maximize their nutrients and minimize the danger of pollutants they may carry.

▶ Remove the skin from fish before cooking it. This won't affect the omega-3 content, but it will lower the overall fat content.

▶ Buy firm, darker species of fish. They often have more omega-3 fats than fish with white flesh.

▶ Shop for fresh finfish — like tuna, trout, cod, snapper, and flounder — that's firm to the touch, has shiny, metallic skin, and no signs of browning or slime. Buy it wrapped in a leakproof package.

▶ Cook fish with moist heat to make the protein in it easier to digest.

Strengthen your immune system with B6

This nutrient knows how to work. It has a hand in building red blood cells, proteins, and even brain chemicals. It regulates your blood sugar and fortifies your immune system.

Lucky for you it's plentiful in protein-rich foods, like fish. That makes it easy to get your quota — 1.5 mg a day for women over age 50 and 1.7 mg for men over age 50. Three ounces of fresh yellowfin tuna gives you about half this recommended amount.

On your off-fish days, be sure to include a variety of B6-rich foods, like bananas, prunes, potatoes, and spinach, or an occasional serving of lean meat, such as turkey or chicken breast.

Fish — benefits outweigh risks

Fish aren't the only ones that suffer from polluted lakes, streams, and oceans. When you serve fish, you also risk eating the toxins they've absorbed. Fish are the main food sources of the toxins mercury and PCBs (polychlorinated biphenyls). The older and larger the fish, the more toxins it may have accumulated. Just how great is the danger? The American Heart Association says the health benefits of eating fish twice a week far outweigh the risks for older men and postmenopausal women.

According to the Food and Drug Administration, most people are safe eating up to 14 ounces a week of fish such as fresh tuna, red snapper, orange roughy, and marlin, which are low in mercury. Wild salmon and mackerel, excellent sources of omega-3s, are virtually free from toxic contaminants. Eat a variety of fish, but avoid long-lived ones, like shark, swordfish, king mackerel, and tilefish.

Reel in better health with vitamin B12

Now that you're supplying your body with all those important omega-3 fatty acids, you need vitamin B12 to put them to good use. This member of the B family also works closely with its cousin, folate, to make red blood cells. What's more, it protects your nerves and is a vital part of many natural body chemicals.

If you're over age 50, your B12 bill totals 2.4 micrograms (mcg) every day. That may not sound like much, but your body has a harder time absorbing it from food as you age. As a result, B12 deficiencies are all too common among older adults. Many health experts recommend you pay close attention to meeting your needs for this nutrient.

Animal foods, particularly fish, shellfish, and red meat, are bursting with B12. Clams, crab, salmon, sardines, trout, and tuna, in particular, are top sources. Fortified cereals add their own share of this vitamin to the mix.

Scientists at Tufts University warn that B12 is one of the few nutrients you may need to supplement as you get older. Nevertheless, always check with your doctor before taking any supplements.

Make zinc your link to wellness

This antioxidant mineral has almost too many jobs to name. It fights free radicals, heals wounds, prevents infections, protects your eyes from macular degeneration, sharpens your sense of taste, and helps your body turn carbohydrates, protein, and fat into energy. Too little zinc in your diet could contribute to poor night vision, lack of appetite, and an impaired sense of taste.

All that work from a tiny amount of zinc. The recommended intake is just 8 mg a day for women over age 50, and 11 mg for men over age 50. Seafood is a treasure trove of zinc. Tuna and sardines supply it in small amounts, but the big contenders are shellfish, like oysters, clams, lobster, shrimp, and crab.

If these foods are a little too rich for your taste, try lean poultry and low-fat dairy products, like yogurt and milk. Many fortified breakfast cereals also pack a zinc punch, so check their Nutrition Facts labels.

In addition to the nutrients you've just read about, fish is also a storehouse of protein and key trace minerals, including selenium, copper, fluoride, and iodine – not to mention major minerals, like calcium, potassium, phosphorus, and magnesium.

The list goes on, but you get the point. Let fish grace your plate two or more times a week, and you'll benefit from its quality nutrition and protective power – important tools you'll need on the road to good health.

Get the most from supplements

You've spent hard-earned money buying high-quality supplements – so protect your investment by storing them properly. Follow these tips from consumer advocate Bill Sardi.

▸ Store supplements in a cool, dark, dry environment. Some vitamins are easily destroyed by light and heat.

▸ Never store your supplements in the refrigerator. The moisture may cause fungal spoilage.

▸ On the road, place them in a hard pill carrier so they don't get squashed in a purse or pocket.

▸ Always use your supplements before their expiration date. If you see brown specks on your pills, it's time to throw them out.`

Week 7

Get the lowdown on nuts, seeds, and meats

For the past six weeks, you've worked on adding wholesome foods to your daily menu. Now, it's time to actively limit certain foods that don't bring the same well-rounded nutrition to your table.

Think of the foods in this group as weekly treats – they all make good nutritional additions when eaten occasionally. Overdoing them, however, could be worse than avoiding them altogether.

Nuts and seeds deliver lots of good-for-you nutrients. A few servings each week could promote heart and joint health. Too many on a regular basis could contribute to weight gain.

Meat also carries both benefits and dangers. This food group includes red meat, poultry, and eggs, mainstays of many Western diets. They are full of saturated fat, which contributes to heart-related health problems. Choose carefully and trim back servings, and you can reduce this risk.

Creating a healthy balance of these foods is your big challenge for week seven, a project you'll take on in two parts. First, you'll learn the game plan for nuts and seeds, and then you'll move on to meat. Practice what you learn and you'll be one step closer to better health.

Squirrel away nutritious nuts and seeds

These tiny but mighty foods can actually protect your health. Studies show if you're a postmenopausal woman, eating nuts frequently may lower your risk of heart disease. And both men and women can cut their risk of dying from a heart attack. The nutrients in seeds, on the other hand, can help treat ailments from cataracts and high cholesterol to osteoarthritis.

Both nuts and seeds are cholesterol-free and jampacked with the antioxidant vitamin E and heart-healthy unsaturated fats. Remember, nuts store lots of energy, meaning they're crammed with calories. That's one reason why a handful here and there could help you stay active, but filling up too often could lead to weight gain.

They are a healthy snack or salad topper, but you don't necessarily need to eat them every day. Just snack on a serving several times during the week to round out your eating plan. One-third cup nuts, one-quarter cup seeds, or two tablespoons nut butter equals one serving.

Nuts and seeds are so small they're easy to forget. In fact, your biggest challenge during week seven may simply be remembering to eat them at all.

Heal your heart with monounsaturated fat

Nuts and seeds are chock-full of an unsaturated fat called monounsaturated fatty acid (MUFA). Like the polyunsaturated fat in fish, MUFAs help put a lid on out-of-control cholesterol and shut out serious illnesses, such as heart disease.

Studies show it doesn't stop there. MUFAs may boost your memory and help prevent high blood pressure, arthritis, diabetes, and some cancers — no small feat.

For extra servings of monounsaturated fat, eat avocados, olives, peanuts, and olive and canola oils. Experts aren't sure exactly how much of this healthy fat you need each day. Instead, they suggest you replace foods high in saturated fat with those rich in MUFAs.

4 easy ways to eat more seeds and nuts

▶ Sprinkle nuts or sunflower seed kernels on salads for a little extra nutrition and flavor.

▶ Dress greens with raw flaxseed oil instead of salad dressings, or drizzle it on cooked vegetables in place of butter.

▶ Toss a few nuts into baked goods or morning meals like pancakes, oatmeal, or cereal.

▶ Try cooking with unusual oils such as walnut or sunflower oil.

Give bad cholesterol the boot with vitamin E

It's added to processed foods to give them a longer shelf life, and vitamin E may do the same for your body. Its anti-aging power comes from a variety of abilities. As an antioxidant, it prevents LDL cholesterol from oxidizing and plaque from building up in your blood vessels. That's good news for your heart health, since that means a lower risk of heart disease and stroke.

As it protects your cells from free radical damage, vitamin E may also protect you from chronic diseases and certain kinds of cancer. It's also linked to mental health and may help your mind stay young as you age. Along with other antioxidants, researchers are hopeful vitamin E could help prevent Alzheimer's disease.

There are four tocopherol, or vitamin E, compounds – alpha, beta, gamma, and delta. Although the most common and powerful form of vitamin E is alpha-tocopherol, many researchers think you should consume all four types, especially gamma-tocopherol.

Good sources of alpha-tocopherol include almonds, olive oil, and sunflower seeds and oil. You'll find gamma-tocopherol in soybean oil and corn oil. Almonds contain alpha-tocopherol and beta-tocopherol, while canola oil has both alpha- and gamma-tocopherol. Wheat germ is a good source of all four types. In general, most sources of unsaturated fats carry a healthy dose of this vitamin.

If you're over the age of 50, you should look for ways to get 15 milligrams of vitamin E each day. You can add more vitamin E by cooking with olive, canola, or corn oils instead of butter or margarine. Just munching a few servings of nuts and seeds each week gives you vitamin E as well as other winning nutrients, such as magnesium, potassium, manganese, chromium and boron, plus vitamins B6, niacin, folate, and thiamin to name a few. Don't forget to make these foods and their oils part of your regular eating habits, and they'll reward you with a longer, healthier life.

It's better to get vitamin E in modest amounts from food than from supplements. Supplements might not offer the same benefits because the vitamin E found in foods is balanced between different kinds of tocopherols. This balance is missing in most vitamin E supplements that contain only a synthetic form of alpha-tocopherol.

What's more, vitamin E is a blood thinner. If you're taking blood thinning medication, like warfarin (Coumadin), taking vitamin E supplements could be dangerous. Studies show taking large doses of vitamin E supplements actually increases death rates.

The truth about meat

Steak, sausage, fried chicken, eggs – foods like these can mean bad news for your heart and your cancer risk. Chosen and prepared carefully, however, meat – including eggs – can be part of a healthy eating plan, just like nuts and seeds. Before you give up on your favorite dish, learn to make it a more wholesome part of your weekly menu. Red meat, poultry, and eggs are stocked with nutrients. They're ripe with protein, loaded with minerals such as phosphorus, selenium, iron, and zinc, and bursting with the vitamins A, B12, thiamin, and niacin.

So what's the beef? Red meat and poultry are also full of saturated fat, the kind that clogs your arteries and contributes to high cholesterol, heart disease, and weight gain. Out of this food group, processed meat, like bacon, and red meats, such as beef, pork, and lamb, may pose the biggest health threat – there's evidence linking them with certain kinds of cancer. Red meat, especially, is loaded with the heme form of iron that may facilitate the growth of cancer cells.

In studying the eating habits of over 100,000 people, experts from Harvard Medical School and the American Cancer Society gave their highest "Healthy Eating" score to people who ate red meat less than twice a month.

Your best bet – make fish your main protein source. Eat fish twice a week, serve poultry occasionally for variety, and limit red meat to two servings each month. A meat serving equals one egg or 2 to 3 ounces of cooked lean meat or skinless poultry. When you include meat in your menu, go for lean cuts, eliminate as much fat as possible – including the skin on poultry – and bake, broil, or grill.

9 ways to reap more benefits

▸ Grind flaxseeds before including them in recipes, and then use them immediately.

▸ Don't fry with flaxseed oil. It breaks down in high heat and could become harmful.

▸ Many kinds of nuts and seeds contain added salt. Check labels, and choose those lowest in sodium if you're salt sensitive.

▸ Check the expiration dates on nut and seed oils, and follow their directions on storing them. Some have short shelf lives.

▸ Substitute a cup of cooked legumes in place of meat twice a week.

▸ Build meals around the plant foods on your plate. Treat meat as just a small part of the larger meal, not the star of it.

▸ Limit meat servings to less than 3 ounces — about the size of a deck of cards.

▸ Gradually cut back meat servings by one-third or even one-half your regular portion at each meal until you reach your serving goal of 2 to 3 ounces.

▸ Choose poultry more often than red meat to satisfy those protein cravings.

Week 8

Sweets and snacks survival guide

You are in the final week of your journey toward better nutrition, and the final change in your diet may surprise you. During week eight, you'll learn to examine all your guilty pleasures – like chips, dips, chocolate, or fries – and determine which ones can stay and which have to go. Amazingly, the news is not all bad.

Snacking can be a healthy habit. It helps maintain steady blood sugar and energy levels to keep you active throughout your day. It's all in what and how much you eat.

Not surprisingly, many sweets and snacks offer little nutrition. Instead, they package sugar, fat, and sodium in a tempting recipe for trouble. That's why many eating plans tell you to give up these goodies completely – a difficult task for even the healthiest eater.

You don't have to forgo your favorite treats on the *Complete Nutrition* eating plan. Just enjoy them in moderation, choosing versions low in sugar, saturated fats, trans fats, and sodium. Learn to weed out the worst of them, find healthy substitutes, and enjoy them as occasional rewards for sticking to your healthy eating plan.

Think 'natural' to satisfy a sweet tooth

Sugar can give fresh fruits their sweet flavor, or sodas their syrupy taste. The difference is in the company it keeps. When you eat fruits or grains, you get a little natural sugar alongside a healthy dose of vitamins, minerals, water, and fiber. Commercial sweets, on the other hand, contain concentrated amounts of refined or added sugar, but few nutrients. You'll get quick energy and little else.

Most of the refined sugar you eat probably comes from processed foods, such as sodas, cakes, cookies, candies, fruit drinks, and dairy desserts, like ice cream. Manufacturers add this extra sugar to tempt your taste buds. Unfortunately, it also contributes to weight gain and tooth decay.

Sweet treats can even edge healthy foods out of your diet. Eating a goody as a reward for hard work isn't a problem for most people.

But indulging your sweet tooth too often can undo the health gains you've made over the last seven weeks.

Although artificial sweeteners, like saccharin and aspartame, sweeten foods without adding extra calories, some research links these sugar substitutes to memory loss, arthritis, migraines, and metabolic syndrome – a group of health problems that occur together, increasing your risk of diabetes, heart attack, and stroke.

Your best bet is to develop a taste for naturally sweet foods – like bananas, strawberries, blueberries, and other delicious fruits – and eat them in place of snack foods high in added sugar.

Surprising link between diet soda and obesity

Just because you drink diet soda doesn't mean you'll lose weight. In fact, you could put yourself at higher risk for metabolic syndrome, a collection of risk factors for heart disease and diabetes.

Recent studies have found a link between the consumption of soda – both regular and diet – and metabolic syndrome. This includes obesity, high cholesterol, high blood pressure, and high blood sugar levels. Similar evidence comes from a study of rats and saccharin, which found that artificial sweeteners caused the rats to eat more and become obese.

One likely explanation is that artificial sweeteners break your body's association between sweet taste and caloric content. Normally, your body gears up to digest more calories when you taste something sweet. When the calories don't follow, you may compensate by eating more. The sweetness of the soda may also lead you to develop a preference for other sweet – and high-calorie – items.

Get the skinny on fats

Junk foods are notoriously high in two types of heart-harming fats — saturated fats and trans fats. A snack made with these bad fats has a longer shelf life than those made with unsaturated fats. That translates into more money for the manufacturers. But if you eat foods full of these fats, your own shelf life could get significantly shorter.

Although it's mostly found in animal foods, like meat and dairy products, saturated fat also shows up in tropical oils — palm, palm kernel, and coconut oils — often used to make snack foods. Surprisingly, coconut oil contains even more saturated fat than pure cream and may significantly raise your risk for heart disease.

Trans fats are different. During processing, manufacturers turn some of a food's unsaturated fat into saturated fat to extend shelf life or change the taste or texture of that food. Trans fatty acids are one of the by-products. The unnatural chemical structure of this "super fat" raises your cholesterol as well as your risk for heart disease and possibly cancer.

Some treats are top suspects for trans and saturated fats. Think twice before eating these:

- most margarines and shortenings

- fast food and fried foods, including chicken, fish, and french fries

- bakery goods, like doughnuts, rolls, biscuits, cakes, and cookies

- chips, corn snacks, and crackers

- salad dressing and mayonnaise

In addition, beware of food with hydrogenated or partially hydrogenated oil in the ingredients list — including many brands of peanut butter. These are code words for trans fats.

> ## 3 smart ways to satisfy a snack attack
>
> ▸ Skip junk food and sugary sodas, and snack on vegetables, whole grains, fruits, and low-fat dairy products instead.
>
> ▸ Serve snacks and treats well before mealtime so you won't ruin your appetite for healthier foods.
>
> ▸ Go easy on portions. Remember, these are snacks, not full meals.

4 golden rules of good nutrition

Don't lose hope if you slip every once in a while and go overboard with your favorite snack or sweet. Just remember the healthy habits you've practiced over the last seven weeks and climb back on your long-life eating plan.

Eating for optimal health is not about going to extremes. It's about getting the nutrients you need and finding a balance in your food lifestyle. You don't have to deprive yourself. You can eat the foods you love and still stay healthy. Just follow the guidelines in your *Complete Nutrition* eating plan and these four golden rules of good nutrition:

▸ Adequacy. Get enough vitamins, minerals, and energy from the food you eat each day to replace what you lose through daily activities.

▸ Moderation. So what if you still love sweets and can't give up red meat. Learn restraint. Enjoy an occasional treat alongside lots of nutritious foods, but monitor unhealthy fats, sugar, and cholesterol.

▸ Balance. While you may have a few favorite foods and food groups, make sure you eat from all of them. For instance, don't ignore calcium-rich foods in favor of those high in iron. You need a healthy balance of nutrients from many different kinds of foods.

▸ Variety. No single food or food group provides all the nutrients you need to stay healthy. Fill your plate with an ever-changing variety of different foods. You'll serve up perfect portions of crucial nutrients and make mealtimes more enjoyable.

Foods are by far the healthiest, most natural way to get quality nutrition. As you age, however, your body's needs change, and you may require more of certain nutrients than you can get from food. According to experts, seniors, in particular, may need more vitamins D and B12, as well as calcium.

Do your best to fill your nutritional needs with food. Still, you might need a multivitamin in addition to a well-rounded eating plan. Always talk with your doctor before taking supplements. Too much of certain vitamins or minerals can be toxic or mask other illnesses and deficiencies.

Caution for people taking Coumadin

Do you eat the same food all year long? Probably not. A bowl of hot chili helps fight the chill of winter. But when the weather warms up, you may prefer cool, fresh salads.

If you are taking the blood thinner Coumadin, a brand of warfarin, this change could be a big mistake. Sudden shifts in your diet may throw off the balance of vitamin K and blood thinners in your system, causing serious problems.

Vitamin K is found in green leafy vegetables, broccoli, canola and soybean oils, and some dietary supplement drinks. It helps your body form clots. Coumadin is prescribed to do the opposite — prevent blood clotting in people at risk for stroke or certain heart problems. Suddenly adding more vitamin K to your diet could change the way the drug works. If you take Coumadin, talk it over with your doctor before changing your diet.

Exercise your heart muscle
Simple steps to a stronger heart

Build a stronger heart for a longer life

Advances in science and technology have given you the opportunity to live longer than ever before. As a 65-year-old, you can expect to live an average of 17.9 more years, much longer than your grandparents ever dreamed of, according to the National Center for Health Statistics.

So what will you do for the next 18 years? Sit and vegetate in your rocking chair or join the active, fun-loving seniors who enjoy life to the fullest? If you want your golden years to burst with vitality, then you need to actively find ways to strengthen your heart and reverse ill health.

That's where fitness fits in. It's not just about firm muscles, endless energy, or a trim waistline. It's about giving your body the weapons it needs to fight off diseases like heart disease and diabetes. If you already have health problems, it's about making the most of your situation.

Up to 300,000 people die each year from diseases or health conditions related to a poor diet and sedentary lifestyle, according to a recent report from the U.S. Department of Health and Human Services. On top of that, inactive lifestyles and unhealthy eating habits may cause as many as 14 out of every 100 deaths in the United States. In fact, sedentary people have double the heart attack risk of those who exercise regularly.

There are four types of exercises, two of which are especially important to fighting heart disease. Most important to maintaining a healthy heart are:

▸ **Endurance or aerobic exercises.** By increasing your breathing and heart rate, these exercises improve the health of your heart, lungs, and circulatory system. Having more endurance improves your stamina for the tasks you need to do to live and do things on your own – climbing stairs and grocery shopping, for example. Endurance exercises also may delay or prevent many diseases associated with aging, such as heart disease and diabetes, and keep you out of the hospital. What's more, regular endurance exercise, like brisk walking, strengthens your immune system, relieves stress, boosts your mood, improves circulation, and lowers blood pressure.

▶ **Strength exercises.** They will help build your muscles, but they do more than just make you stronger. They give you more strength to do things on your own. Even very small increases in muscle can make a big difference in ability, especially for frail people. Strength exercises also increase your metabolism, helping to keep your weight and blood sugar in check. That's important because obesity and diabetes are major health problems for older adults. Studies suggest strength exercises also may help prevent osteoporosis.

The other types of exercises affect balance and flexibility. Balance exercises help prevent falls, a common problem in older adults. Falling is a major cause of broken hips and other injuries that often lead to disability and loss of independence. Some balance exercises also build up your leg muscles. Flexibility exercises help keep your body limber by stretching your muscles and the tissues that hold your body's structures in place.

Physical therapists and other health professionals recommend certain stretching exercises to help people recover from injuries and to prevent injuries from ever happening. Flexibility also may play a part in preventing falls.

Rediscover youthful energy. But here's some good news. Every time you exercise, you may be one step closer to saving your heart – or even your life. So why wait? You can grow younger in just about every measurable way – including your appearance, health, energy, and memory – by adopting healthy habits and a "can-do" attitude.

The first thing exercise does is boost your endurance and give you new energy. If you often feel exhausted, lack of exercise could be a factor. Think about it. When you don't exercise your muscles and your other body parts, they aren't as well conditioned to handle physical demands. Not surprisingly, that leads you to wear out more quickly. Scientists have nicknamed this problem "sedentary inertia."

But exercise can be the answer — if you stay with it long enough. At first, the extra action will make you more tired because it places new demands on your body. On the other hand, you may sleep more soundly, too. Over time, your body will grow stronger and get used to this new level of activity. One day, you could suddenly realize you have more energy than you used to — and a lot more stamina.

Fascinating fact

Together, lack of exercise and poor diet are the second-largest underlying cause of death in the United States. Smoking is the #1 cause.

Exercise makes you 'young-at-heart'

You're never "too old" and "too frail" to exercise. In fact, there aren't very many health reasons to keep you from becoming more active. It's a good idea to get your doctor's approval before starting an exercise program. Your doctor can talk to you not only about whether it's all right for you to exercise but also about what can be gained from exercise.

Exercise is the new Rx. Chronic diseases, like cardiovascular disease and diabetes, may not be curable, but usually they can be controlled or improved with medications and other treatments. In the past, exercise has been discouraged in people with certain chronic conditions. But researchers have found that exercise can actually improve some chronic conditions in older people, as long as it's done when the condition is under control.

Congestive heart failure (CHF) is an example of a serious chronic condition common in older adults. In people with CHF, the heart can't empty its load of blood with each beat, resulting in a backup of fluid throughout the body, including the lungs. Heart rhythm disturbances also are common in CHF. Older adults are hospitalized more often for this disease than for any other.

No one is sure why, but muscles tend to waste away badly in people with CHF, leaving them weak, sometimes to the point that they can't perform everyday tasks. No medicine has a direct muscle-strengthening effect in people with CHF, but muscle-building exercises, like lifting weights, can help improve muscle strength.

Having a chronic disease, like CHF, probably doesn't mean you can't exercise, but it does mean you should talk with your doctor before exercising. For example, some studies suggest endurance exercises, like brisk walking, may improve how well the heart and lungs work in people with CHF, but only in people who are in a stable phase of the disease.

People with CHF, like those with most chronic diseases, have periods when their disease gets better, then worse, then better again, off and on. The same endurance exercises that might help people in a stable phase of CHF could be very harmful to people who are in an unstable phase, when they have fluid in their lungs or an irregular heart rhythm.

Know your stage. If you have a chronic condition, you need to know whether your disease is stable and if exercise will benefit you. Talk with your doctor about symptoms that mean trouble – a flare-up, or what doctors call an acute phase or exacerbation of your disease. If you have CHF, you know by now the acute phase of this disease should be taken seriously. You should not exercise when warning symptoms of the acute phase of any chronic disease appear.

Lower heart-damaging high blood sugar. Diabetes is another chronic condition common among older people and linked to heart disease. Too much sugar in the blood is a hallmark of diabetes. It can cause damage throughout the body. Exercise can help your body "use up" some of the damaging sugar. The most common form of diabetes is linked to physical inactivity.

In other words, you are less likely to get it if you stay physically active. If you have diabetes and it has caused changes in your body — cardiovascular disease, eye disease, or changes in your nervous system, for example — check with your doctor to find out what exercises will help you and whether you should avoid certain activities. If you take insulin or a pill that helps lower your blood sugar, your doctor might need to adjust your dose as you start to exercise so your blood sugar doesn't get too low.

Keep your doctor informed. Check with your doctor first if you plan to start doing vigorous physical activities, which could be a problem for people who have "hidden" heart disease — when people are unaware of their heart disease because they don't have any symptoms. How can you tell if the activity you plan to do is vigorous? There are a couple of ways. If the activity makes you breathe hard and sweat hard, you can consider it vigorous.

Charts later in this chapter explain more about how to tell if your exercise is moderate or vigorous. If you have had a heart attack recently, your doctor or cardiac rehabilitation therapist should have given you specific exercises to do. Research has shown that exercises done as part of a cardiac rehabilitation program can improve fitness and even reduce your risk of dying.

Be sure to check with your doctor before beginning any kind of exercise program if you have either an abdominal aortic aneurysm, a weakness in the wall of the heart's major outgoing artery, or critical aortic stenosis, a narrowing of one of the valves of the heart. Most older adults, regardless of age or condition, will do fine if they increase their physical activity.

Exercise checkpoints

You have already read about precautions you should take if you have a chronic condition. Other circumstances require caution, too. You shouldn't exercise until checking with a doctor if you have:

▸ chest pain

▸ irregular, rapid, or fluttery heartbeat

▸ severe shortness of breath

▸ significant, ongoing weight loss that hasn't been diagnosed

▸ infections, such as pneumonia, accompanied by fever

▸ fever, which can cause dehydration and a rapid heartbeat

▸ acute deep-vein thrombosis (blood clot)

▸ a hernia that is causing symptoms

▸ foot or ankle sores that won't heal

▸ joint swelling

▸ persistent pain or a problem walking after you have fallen

▸ certain eye conditions, such as bleeding in the retina or detached retina

▸ recently undergone cataract or lens implant – or other eye surgery

Endurance-level exercise benefits heart

An easy exercise for one person might be strenuous for another. Listen to your body to know how hard you should exercise. Your estimation of the level of effort you are putting into an activity is probably accurate when compared with physical measurements, according to scientific research. In other words, if you think you are moderately exercising your body, measurements of how hard your heart is working would probably show moderate exertion. During moderate activity, you can sense you are challenging yourself, but you aren't near your limit.

One way you can estimate how hard to work is by using The Borg Category Rating Scale, named after the scientist who developed it. The numbers on the left of the scale help you describe how hard you feel you are working.

For endurance or aerobic activities, you should gradually work your way up to level 13 – the feeling that you are working at a somewhat hard level. Some people might feel that way when they are walking on flat ground. Others, when they are jogging up a hill. Both are right. Only you know how hard your exercise feels to you.

Once you start exerting more than a moderate amount of effort in your cardio-building exercises, your endurance is likely to increase quickly. As your body adapts and you become more fit, you can gradually keep making your activities more challenging.

You might find, for example, that walking on a flat surface used to feel like you were working at level 13 on the Borg scale, but now you have to walk up a mild hill to feel like you are working at level 13. Later, you might find you need to walk up an even steeper slope to feel you are working at level 13.

Check with a fitness professional if you think you are doing the exercises correctly, but you aren't progressing or you are exhausted by your effort. You may not be estimating your effort correctly. Fitness experts can teach you how to match your level of effort with the right number on the Borg scale.

The Borg Category Rating Scale

Least effort

6

7 very, very light

8

9 very light

10

11 fairly light

12   **Endurance Training Zone**

13 somewhat hard

14

15 hard

16

17 very hard

18

19 very, very hard

20

Maximum effort

Improve your endurance with exercise

Endurance exercises are any activity – walking, jogging, swimming, raking – that increases your heart rate and breathing for an extended period of time. Here's how you can get the most from these exercises.

▸ Build up your endurance gradually, starting out with as little as five minutes of endurance activities at a time, if you need to.

▸ Starting out at a lower level of effort and working your way up gradually is especially important if you have been inactive for a long time. It may take months to go from a very long-standing sedentary lifestyle to doing endurance-level training.

▸ Your goal is to work your way up, eventually, to a moderate-to-vigorous level that increases your breathing and heart rate. It should feel somewhat hard to you – level 13 on the Borg scale.

▸ Once you reach your goal, you can divide your exercise into sessions of 10 minutes at a time, if you want to, as long as they add up to a minimum of 30 minutes at the end of the day. Doing less than 10 minutes at a time won't give you the desired cardiovascular and respiratory system benefits. The exception to this guideline is when you are just beginning to do endurance activities.

▸ Your goal is to build up to a minimum of 30 minutes of endurance exercise on most or all days of the week. More often is better, and every day is best.

▸ Endurance activities should not make you breathe so hard you can't talk. They should not cause dizziness or chest pain.

▸ Do a little light activity, like easy walking, before and after your endurance exercise session to warm up and cool down.

▶ Stretch after your endurance activities, when your muscles are warm.

▶ As you get older, your body may become less likely to trigger the urge to drink when you need water. In other words, you may need water, but you won't feel thirsty. Be sure to drink liquids when you are doing any activity that makes you lose fluid through sweat. By the time you notice you are thirsty, you are already somewhat dehydrated or low on fluid. This guideline is important year-round, but it is especially important in hot weather, when dehydration is more likely. If your doctor has asked you to limit your fluids, be sure to check with him before increasing the amount of fluid you drink while exercising. Congestive heart failure and kidney disease are examples of chronic diseases that often require fluid restriction.

▶ Older adults can be affected by heat and cold more than other adults. In extreme cases, exposure to too much heat can cause heatstroke, and exposure to very cold temperatures can lead to hypothermia – a dangerous drop in body temperature. If you are exercising outdoors, dress in layers so you can add or remove clothes as needed.

▶ Use safety equipment to prevent injuries. For example, wear a helmet for bicycling, and wear protective equipment for activities like skiing and skating. If you walk or jog, wear stable shoes made for that purpose.

When you are ready to progress, build up the amount of time you spend doing endurance activities and then build up the difficulty of your activities later. Gradually increase your time to 30 minutes over several weeks or months by walking longer distances, then start walking up steeper hills or walking more briskly.

Tips on how to gauge your effort

Here are some informal guidelines you can use to estimate how much effort you are putting into your endurance activities.

▶ Talking doesn't take much effort during moderate activity. During vigorous activity, talking is difficult.

▶ If you tend to perspire, you probably won't sweat during light activity, except on hot days. You will sweat during vigorous or sustained moderate activity.

▶ Your muscles may get a rubbery feeling after vigorous activity, but not after moderate activity.

▶ One doctor who specializes in exercise for older adults tells her patients this about how hard they should work during endurance activities: "If you can't talk while you're exercising, it's too difficult. If you can sing a song from an opera, it's too easy!"

Examples of endurance activities

Examples of moderate and vigorous activities for the typical older adult are listed below and on the following page.

Moderate:

▶ swimming

▶ bicycling

▶ cycling on a stationary bicycle

▶ gardening (mowing, raking)

▶ walking briskly on a level surface

▶ mopping or scrubbing floor

▶ golf, without a cart

▶ tennis (doubles)

▶ volleyball

▶ rowing

▶ dancing

Vigorous:

▶ climbing stairs or hills

▶ shoveling snow

▶ brisk bicycling up hills

▶ tennis (singles)

▶ swimming laps

▶ cross-country skiing

▶ downhill skiing

▶ hiking

▶ jogging

Unbeatable way to reach your target

Some people use something called a target heart rate to make sure they exercise hard enough, instead of the Borg scale. Yet, some medications and conditions affect your heart rate (HR) and, therefore, interfere with this type of measurement. If you'd like to track your fitness efforts using your target heart rate, get your doctor's approval first.

According to the American Heart Association, your target heart rate range should fall between 50 percent and 75 percent of your maximum heart rate. People with heart risk factors, like high blood pressure, diabetes, high cholesterol, or obesity, should stay between 55 percent and 75 percent. If you've been inactive, first try for 50 percent to 60 percent. For top-notch results, maintain your target heart rate for at least 20 minutes.

If your doctor approves, start exercising at 50 percent of your maximum heart rate. Over several weeks, gradually increase how hard you exercise until you reach 75 percent of your maximum heart rate. For example, if you're 55 years old, you'd start near a target heart rate of 83 beats per minute and eventually work up to around 123. See the chart on page 229 to determine your target heart rate.

If you're at a low fitness level, you may need to work below 50 percent of your target heart rate at first. You can gradually work up to the 50-percent level, then move on to higher levels in your range. You should never reach your maximum heart rate. In fact, do not try to push yourself up beyond 75 percent without checking with your doctor. If you're not already very physically fit, levels above 75 percent could be dangerous. Call your doctor if you have the following symptoms. You may be in danger from exercising too vigorously.

▶ dizziness

▶ difficulty breathing

▶ nausea

▶ pain in your chest, back, left shoulder or arm

If you experience joint pain, extreme fatigue, or problems sleeping, check with your doctor.

Target heart rates during exercise

Age	50% of max HR (beats per minute)	75% of max HR (beats per minute)	Maximum HR
40	90	135	180
45	88	131	175
50	85	127	170
55	83	123	165
60	80	120	160
65	78	116	155
70	75	113	150

Sidestep deadly diseases

Use fitness as your weapon against aging, and you may also fend off the dangerous health problems associated with growing older. In fact, it may be easier than you think. Consider these examples from scientific and medical studies.

▶ Walk 30 to 45 minutes three times a week, and you can cut your risk of heart attack in half.

▶ Slash your odds of type 2 diabetes by 50 percent with just 40 minutes of moderate exercise each week.

▶ Exercise may be as effective as medication at increasing good cholesterol levels and reducing the bad. That means healthier arteries, lower blood pressure, and a lower risk of stroke and heart disease.

▶ Regular physical activity can help people who already suffer from arthritis, depression, heart disease, high blood pressure, high cholesterol, diabetes, osteoporosis, or excess weight.

▶ Being fit may also give you the fortitude to help fight cancer.

Slash your risk of stroke by 80 percent

A British study of people who continued vigorous exercise from ages 15 to 55 had an 80 percent less chance of having a stroke than non-exercisers.

Follow these important steps on the quest for a healthier you.

▸ Pick an exercise that fits your budget and lifestyle.

▸ Consider hiring a trainer for a one-on-one session to make sure you're doing everything right.

▸ Take a class.

▸ Start small. Plan three 10-minute sessions throughout the day.

▸ Stretch.

▸ Raise your heart rate to a safe level. Talk to your doctor about your target heart rate.

▸ Get extra motivation from an exercise group or buddy.

▸ Stop exercising and consult your doctor if you experience joint pain; extreme fatigue; dizziness; difficulty breathing; nausea; or chest, arm, or shoulder pain.

3 ways to get more gusto from your walk

Walking is a fun, cheap, and relatively easy form of exercise. You don't need extensive training to get started, and your heart and lungs benefit from the activity.

Want to lower your risk of stroke? Walking may be the answer. A new study found you don't need to run a marathon to improve your outlook. Walking just three blocks a day lowered stroke risk 30 percent, and walking a mile (about five blocks) cut risk in half for men between the ages of 50 and 60 years. This seems to be true even if you smoke or have high blood pressure or diabetes, say researchers. Imagine how much good walking can do for you if you don't have those other risk factors.

Walking doesn't require any special talent or training – you just do it without thinking. Yet, if you put a little extra time and effort into it each day, just look at the results. You lose weight, have more energy, lower your blood pressure and cholesterol, think more clearly, have less anxiety, and sleep a whole lot better. And that's just the beginning.

Set a goal. You may feel good enough to start out with 20-minute sessions, but if not, that's all right. Just pick a starting point and keep going farther and faster until you get where you want to be. Stick to your starting pace for a week and then start walking a little longer.

Make a 20-minute walk your first goal. That's about how long it takes to start getting real endurance benefits from sustained exercise. A good rule of thumb is to step it up about 10 percent a week. The chart on page 233 shows a schedule to get from 15 minutes to 45 minutes in about three months. This program works best when you're walking about five days a week. If you're walking fewer than three days a week, you should increase your time more slowly.

Pace yourself. If you walk a mile in 20 minutes, you're going 3 miles per hour (mph), which is a low-end moderate pace. Don't worry if you're only doing 2 or 2 1/2 mph. Your exertion level is what's important. Don't overdo it. As your stamina improves, you will naturally speed up just to maintain your heart rate.

So far, you've been working to build up your walking time, but as you get into better shape, you can also raise your exertion level.

Walk faster to boost your heartbeat a little more. Be careful that you don't increase both your speed and walking time during the same workout. Increase one first, then the other a day or two later. Make it your next goal to do three miles in 45 minutes — a 4-mph pace — and then keep going until you top out with a heart rate around 75 percent of your maximum.

A brisk pace is important. If you're not sweating and breathing harder than normal, you're not getting a good workout. Don't stroll or saunter, but don't go too fast, or you'll wear out too soon. Use the "talk test" to find the right pace – slow down if you can't carry on a conversation while you walk.

How long and how hard you walk is much more meaningful than how far you walk. At the top of the list is how often you walk. If you don't walk regularly, you won't see steady improvement, and you can even lose ground. Walk at least three times a week to maintain a general level of fitness. Walk more often if you want to lose weight or raise your endurance level. But always schedule at least one day of rest per week. Your body needs some "down time" to recover.

Focus on good form. Any new exercise program may cause a few aches and pains, but they shouldn't last. Use good technique as you walk, and you'll feel better as if by magic.

▶ Keep your chin up, your shoulders back, and your belly flat.

▶ Take long, easy strides and land on your heel, rolling forward to the ball of your foot and pushing off from the toe.

▶ Breathe deeply and let your arms swing naturally.

▶ Lean forward a little when going fast or up and down hills.

	Warm up	Brisk walk	Cool down	Total time
Walking plan – 45 minutes in 12 weeks				
Week 1	5 min	5 min	5 min	15 min
Week 2	5 min	7 min	5 min	17 min
Week 3	5 min	9 min	5 min	19 min
Week 4	5 min	11 min	5 min	21 min
Week 5	5 min	13 min	5 min	23 min
Week 6	5 min	15 min	5 min	25 min
Week 7	5 min	18 min	5 min	28 min
Week 8	5 min	21 min	5 min	31 min
Week 9	5 min	24 min	5 min	34 min
Week 10	5 min	27 min	5 min	37 min
Week 11	5 min	31 min	5 min	41 min
Week 12	5 min	35 min	5 min	45 min

Every step helps your heart

Some people think walking is too easy to be good exercise. Others believe you can have "gain without pain," and running and jogging are too hard on your body. The fact is, you burn just as many calories per mile walking as you do running. It just takes longer – 20 minutes to walk a mile versus eight or 10 minutes to jog it. A Harvard study found that walking protects you from heart problems just as much as more vigorous and challenging exercise.

Since it's also true that walkers suffer fewer injuries, you may as well walk if you have the time. It's important to walk briskly. You won't experience conditioning or weight loss unless you raise your heart rate.

If you don't have time to walk regularly, try turning your whole day into a series of mini-workouts. You probably do a lot of walking already without even thinking about it. The average adult takes 3,000 to 5,000 steps each day. If you punch that number up to 10,000, experts say, you'll get the equivalent of a steady 30-minute workout. Fitness experts in Japan first tried out the idea, and now it has caught on in America. Researchers at Stanford University and at the Cooper Institute in Dallas have researched it and agree it seems to work.

You can reach 10,000 steps by literally counting every step you take. Rebecca Lindbergh of Health Partners, a managed care organization in Minnesota, coordinates a program in which people actually wear a pedometer to tally their walking. "We encourage them to wear the pedometer all day long," she says about her participants. "They use the pedometer and slip activity in throughout their day." For example, you can:

- ▶ Park farther away at the mall.

- ▶ Take the stairs instead of the escalator.

- ▶ Walk the golf course instead of taking a cart.

- ▶ Spend your coffee break on a walk instead of standing around the water cooler.

- ▶ March through your local mall, and browse every store that catches your fancy.

- ▶ Walk while you're on the phone or during television commercial breaks.

With a pedometer, you begin to notice how these little changes add up to more and more steps. "Using a pedometer puts a little pizzazz into walking," Lindbergh notes. "It's very eye-opening." If you would like to count 10,000 steps, you can find a pedometer at any sporting goods store. If you don't want to spring for one, just try to fit lots of steps into your day in as many ways as possible.

Join the ranks of well-known walkers

Walking is a popular fitness activity, but it's not a new pursuit. Famous walkers throughout history include Harry Truman, noted for his morning presidential walks, and writers Emerson and Thoreau, who walked for inspiration.

Fun way to flatten your belly

One of the risk factors for heart disease is excess fat around the middle of the body, or being apple-shaped. Here's a way to fight that fat and strengthen and tone your stomach. You don't need to do gut-wrenching exercises to turn ugly flab into rock-hard abs. Just get on a giant, inflatable ball called an exercise ball – or a stability, Swiss, physio, or Sissel ball.

The latest rage is to do crunches on an exercise ball. You can now abandon sit-ups for the less demanding but more effective curl-up or crunch. It's an easy exercise to flatten your bulging belly and strengthen your back and stomach muscles.

Physical therapists from Germany and Switzerland have long used the balls for sports training and rehabilitation. Many therapeutic and athletic-conditioning professionals have used these "Swiss balls" since the late 1980s. Today they are a staple for personal trainers and health clubs.

How it works. Crunches aren't the only exercises that can be done with the balls. They are used for everything from push-ups to calf stretches to strength training. Most exercises involve sitting or lying on the ball, either face up or face down.

The ball's key advantage for exercise is its instability. The ball requires you to balance yourself while exercising, which forces you to use a variety of muscles, particularly in the "core" area of your abdomen, back, and hips.

So while you're working out your arms or legs, you're also strengthening these important parts of your body. Core conditioning helps prevent back pain and other injuries and allows you to perform everyday activities more easily. More importantly, belly fat – the abdominal fat that makes your waist large and gives you an apple-shaped body – raises your risk for heart disease, diabetes, and other health problems.

What the experts say. Does the ball help increase your fitness level? Training journals and press releases suggest considerable benefits, but scientific evidence isn't quite as enthusiastic. Here's what studies have shown.

▶ Abdominal muscles get a better workout when crunches are done on exercise balls.

▶ Rugby players who trained with exercise balls suffered fewer low back and groin injuries.

▶ Swimmers and runners improved their core stability but didn't improve their race times.

The general conclusion is that you're not going to get stronger arms and legs from instability training, but you can get a stronger torso – core stability – and better balance and posture.

Before you begin. There are a number of exercises you can do on an exercise ball, but a great many are designed for physical therapy rehabilitation or training for athletic events. The difficulty level can be adjusted by changing either the exercise or the air pressure in the ball. It helps to begin by working with an experienced trainer.

Normal fitness benefits from these balls relate mostly to abdominal training. Not surprisingly, improved muscle tone in your abs helps with everyday tasks and prevents back pain. But it's best to get some experience with an exercise on solid ground before you do it on an exercise ball.

Amazing 'side effect' of exercise

Exercise is one of the best ways to lose weight and lower your blood pressure. Now research reveals even more good news. The study found blood pressure was lower even hours after exercising. After three 15-minute sessions on a treadmill, men had reductions in systolic blood pressure that lasted for 16 hours. Reductions in diastolic blood pressure remained for 12 hours.

Average blood pressure readings were lower overall for the 24-hour period following exercise than on days when the men didn't exercise. This means your heart doesn't have to work quite as hard for hours after you exercise. So give your heart a break and take a hike, go for a walk, fly a kite — just move it.

If you have uncontrolled high blood pressure or are older, be careful about starting vigorous exercise. You may be at a slightly higher risk for a heart attack. Check with your doctor.

Reap big rewards in just 11 minutes twice a day

Like an unexpected care package, exercise can be full of pleasant surprises. Physical activity is packed with perks that can make you happier and healthier. In fact, the list of benefits is so long it's impossible to include everything, but here are a few examples.

Fights fatigue. You might think you don't have the energy to exercise now that you're older, but exercise will actually give you a natural energy boost. Even a 10-minute workout may foil fatigue, because it releases chemicals in your brain that improve your mood. Make physical activity a regular part of your day, and you could soon feel as peppy as a 25-year-old.

If that natural energy boost from getting active isn't enough, exercise also improves your ability to fall asleep and sleep well. So if lack of sleep is the reason your get-up-and-go has gotten up and went, a little physical activity could have you feeling more energetic.

Add some relaxation techniques to your physical activity and you'll feel even better. Spending a minute doing deep breathing can slow your heart rate, lower your blood pressure, improve digestion, and regulate your blood sugar. Try this quick routine.

▶ Get comfortable, either sitting or lying down. Remind yourself to inhale through your nose and exhale through your mouth.

▶ Slowly exhale, pushing most of the air out of your lungs.

▶ Inhale slowly while you count to four. Breathe into your belly and don't lift your shoulders. As you breathe, think about the air's warmth flowing throughout your body.

▶ Pause for a second, then slowly exhale while you count to four. Imagine the stress draining out of your body along with the air.

▶ Continue breathing deeply until you feel calm.

Practice your physical fitness and stress-reduction routine every morning and evening.

Fends off deadly diseases. Heart disease, stroke, cancer, and diabetes are dangerous, devastating conditions. Yet, physical activity can help fight them all. For instance, walk 30 to 45 minutes three times a week and cut your heart attack risk in half. That's right — time spent walking rather than distance covered is what's important. Here's what else exercise can do for heart health.

▶ reduce the risk of a second heart attack

▶ cut triglycerides and total cholesterol

▶ lower the risk of developing high blood pressure

▶ keep resting blood pressure rates lower for hours after an exercise session ends

▶ shrink your chances of developing and dying from heart disease

Boosts your brainpower. Aerobic exercise feeds your brain cells with oxygen and nutrients. That may be why physical activity can encourage creativity and speed your thinking. Exercise can also tighten up your reaction time and help you process information faster.

With your brain working at full capacity, you have a better chance of solving problems and making well-reasoned decisions. Fascinating new research finds physical activity may ward off Alzheimer's disease, one of the most dreaded senior diseases. Exercise increases brain chemicals that help the growth of new brain nerve cells. Dr. Susan Spalding, a Certified Movement Analyst, is Director of Dance Programs at Berea College in Kentucky. She explains why dancing — such as square dancing or contra dancing — might give you a leg up on brainpower.

"It helps memory because of the complex coordinations involved," she says. "It helps with both short-term and long-term memory, and has been recommended as a defense against Alzheimer's disease."

A study out of Case Western Reserve University School of Medicine in Ohio supports the theory that regular exercise – especially between the ages of 20 and 60 years – may lower your chances of getting Alzheimer's disease. Experts emphasize that you must exercise over the long-term to do any good.

Dance your way to a happy heart

Waltz, tango, swing, two-step – they're all fun dances that get your body moving and your heart pumping. Researchers in Italy studied dance as exercise for people with moderate heart failure. They compared those who walked on treadmills and rode stationary bikes three times a week with people who waltzed with a partner for at least 20 minutes three times a week. People in a third group got no exercise.

After two months, people who exercised had better heart and lung health than those in the sedentary group. That's no surprise. But the researchers were startled to find that dancing seemed to create a bigger improvement in happiness and quality of life. So grab a partner and put on your dancing shoes.

Guaranteed weight-loss secret

Watching your weight usually involves focusing on what you eat. But don't overlook the other key part of any successful weight-loss program. If you want to shed pounds, you not only have to take in fewer calories – you also have to burn more. That means exercising.

Regular exercise does so much more than just help you lose weight. You can reduce blood pressure and cholesterol, relieve chronic pain and anxiety, and lower your medical bills all with one simple self-help method. So get moving.

Step lively. Don't worry. Exercising doesn't have to include heavy weights, long runs, or fancy machines. A brisk 30-minute walk every day will help. So will everyday activities, such as raking, gardening, or cleaning up around your house. Anything that gives you a workout counts as exercise.

Spread it out. If you can't spend 30 minutes exercising, split your exercise time into three 10-minute sessions or two 15-minute ones. Short bursts of exercise work just as well as one longer session when it comes to burning calories and losing weight.

Try something new. Looking for a change? If you're tired of walking or lifting weights, think about the fun sports that keep you moving. Swimming, tennis, bicycling, golf, and stair walking are all good ways to keep fit. Make sure you talk to your doctor before you begin a new exercise program.

Best dieting tool — heart-healthy exercise

Dieting is well and good, but to lose weight and keep it off, you must exercise, too. That's your secret weapon. The more muscle you have, the more calories you'll burn – even when you're just watching TV. Cutting back on calories without exercising leads to bone loss in your hips and spine. Try this advice to supercharge your workouts and help those pounds melt away.

Invest in weights. Strength training halts the middle-age spread of your waistline. It builds muscle, which in turn helps you burn more calories – even while you sleep. In fact, a study showed that overweight, middle-age women who lifted weights just twice a week became stronger and did not gain weight as they aged, the opposite of what happens to most people. In particular, these women lost belly fat, which lowered their risk of heart disease.

Your muscles need new challenges to keep growing, much like your brain. Alternate which muscles you work each day – legs one day, arms and back the next – and avoid working the same ones two days in a row. Gradually add more repetitions and increase the amount of weight you lift.

Get your heart pumping. The heart is a muscle, too. Keep it in tip-top shape with aerobic activities that get your heart rate up, like brisk walking, dancing, and swimming. Swap out activities regularly. If you swim one day, then walk or jog the next. Boost the benefit even more by slowing down for five minutes, then speeding up for five minutes.

Women trying to lose weight should aim for a moderate – but not intense – endurance or aerobic workout. Strenuous activity actually stimulates women's appetites, prompting them to eat more. Moderate activity doesn't. In one study, women who did moderate aerobic workouts lost more weight than those who trained intensely. Men don't have this problem. The harder they exercise, the more calories they burn.

Do something you enjoy. Working out doesn't have to mean gym memberships and aerobic classes. It can mean yard work, yoga, and a daily walk. Find an exercise you enjoy or one that makes you feel accomplished, then stick with it until it becomes habit. Your body and mind will get "addicted" in a good way, and you won't want to miss a day.

Keep moving. Exercise will only do so much. If you walk for 30 minutes but spend the rest of the day watching TV, you won't lose weight. It's fine to relax, but stay active throughout the day as much as possible to maximize your weight loss. You'll drop those pounds in no time.

> ## Smart way to save money on medical bills
>
> Exercise saves you money. According to a survey, active Americans older than 15 years saved an annual average of $330 in medical costs compared to people who were inactive. Consider fitness your personal savings plan.

Lower blood pressure with gentle tai chi

Looking for a change in your exercise program? Try tai chi. This traditional Chinese exercise program is perfect for older people. It improves your balance, cardiovascular fitness, and your ability to walk, lift things, and even run.

You can practice tai chi indoors or out, alone or in a group, and its gentle movements make it ideal for people who want a workout but whose bones can't take the jarring that comes with many forms of exercise.

Tai chi is an ancient form of exercise that involves a series of slow, concentrated movements designed to take you through a wide range of motion over a prolonged period of time – 10 to 60 minutes.

Seniors who practiced it 30 minutes a day, four days a week for 12 weeks, reduced their blood pressure about as much as those in a more strenuous aerobic exercise program. Experts say tai chi is a safe, beneficial exercise choice for people after a heart attack. It's also an effective activity to help lower your blood pressure.

As with most inner arts, there is much more to tai chi than meets the eye. It offers both physical and mental benefits. Physically, you must use the strength of your lower body to support your fluid movement. Then you must work on your balance whenever you step or kick. At the same time, your upper-body flexibility is improved by doing the smooth, even movements.

Overall coordination is improved just by trying to get upper-body movements synchronized with lower-body movements. In fact, long-term studies on older people who practice tai chi have found they have better heart and lung function, flexibility, balance, muscle strength, and endurance — along with less body fat — than inactive people.

Tai chi is more than just a physical challenge, however. It's also a great mental exercise, requiring you to learn the order of the movements, remember what direction you should be facing at all times, pay attention to where your weight is, and plan where you will move next. Finally, the deliberate motions and intense focus may help you relax. To perform tai chi well, you must be calm and "present" in the moment, leaving your other worries or concerns behind.

Be sure to find a knowledgeable teacher who can teach you tai chi correctly. It's usually taught in martial arts schools and often in community centers, adult-education classes, fitness centers, or YMCAs. Also, the Arthritis Foundation has an exercise program based on tai chi called ROM (range of motion) dance.

Once you learn the movements, tai chi can be deeply gratifying. It is an art or discipline you can practice in a small space. It requires no special clothing or equipment, and it can be satisfying no matter how much or how little time is available.

Cycling your way to a better heart

In 1973, John Karras and Don Kaul, both writers for *The Des Moines Register*, decided to ride bicycles from one end of Iowa to the other producing columns and articles for the newspaper along the way. They invited their readers to join them, and between 100 and 500 riders cycled in and out of the six-day ride.

The event was so successful that it turned into RAGBRAI – the Register's Annual Great Bicycle Ride Across Iowa – and now must limit the number of weeklong riders to 8,500. It has also inspired more than 40 similar rides around the country. Karras rode in 28 events and wrote stories about the trip and the towns they went through, traveling 450 to 500 miles, fighting hills, heat, humidity, and headwinds.

"I bought my first 10-speed bicycle in 1967 at age 37, and it changed my life," Karras recalls. "I had ridden some as a child and a lot the summers of my college years – all on an old one-speed, fat-tired bike. The 10-speed was a revelation. I thought I'd never have to pedal again. I talked my best friend into buying one, and in a few years, we had become touring cyclists, discovering that Iowa is incredibly beautiful from the seat of a bicycle. The more we rode, the fitter we became."

Neither had been athletes as young men, but the bikes changed all that. Now 73 and retired in Colorado, Karras is no longer an official part of RAGBRAI, but he and his wife, Ann, still bike, hike, and ski.

"How fit am I?" Karras asks. "Compared to the general population of my age, very. Compared to the seniors in Summit County, maybe average or a little below. We live above 9,000 feet, which makes just about everything a little more difficult. Last year, for the first time since we moved here, we approached our old levels of fitness. We managed to ride about 1,500 miles."

If riding a bike sounds like a great way for you to get fit, follow this advice, and you'll be cycling in no time.

Karras's story demonstrates the appeal bicycling has for many people. It's one of America's most popular activities and one of the best aerobic exercises. But you don't have to ride 4,000 miles a year as Karras and his wife used to do for fun and fitness from your two-wheeler.

Simply pedal around your neighborhood – get your heart pumping a little faster for 20 or 30 minutes and enjoy the sights you never see from a car window.

If you are lucky, you can take a trail ride through nearby parks. Why not ride your bike to work, particularly if you live where traffic and parking are frustrating? If biking becomes a passion, consider a newer bike – they now come with up to 30 speeds – and venture into the country for day trips.

However you ride, you are steadily and continuously working your large lower-body muscles. This prompts your heart and lungs to carry more oxygen, increasing your overall fitness.

Lighten up
Secrets to winning the battle of the bulge

Say goodbye to extra pounds for good

More than a billion people in the world are either obese or over-weight, and the numbers are expanding rapidly. Excess weight boosts your risk of serious diseases, some of them deadly. Obesity costs Americans more than $117 billion every year in medical costs and lost productivity.

Weight gain is not a mystery. When you put more fuel – or food – into your body than you burn, the excess energy is stored as fat. To manage your weight, you must balance energy intake with output.

The search is always on for a quick and easy solution – a miracle diet, magic pill, or super exercise machine. But in the end, the only proven solution is a combination of sensible eating habits and regular physical activity.

Add years to your life. You look good and feel energetic when you maintain a trim figure, but your health is an even more important reason to watch your weight. Doctors used to think after age 55 people didn't gain and, in fact, gradually lost pounds. But that doesn't hold true. Obesity, or excess body fat, is growing faster among seniors than any other group.

Experts say extra weight hurts your health even more than smoking or heavy drinking. It increases your risk for diabetes, heart disease, stroke, high blood pressure, gallbladder disease, sleep apnea and other breathing problems, osteoarthritis, and some forms of cancer. But the good news is, you can do something about it.

If you are overweight, starting on a healthy weight-loss plan now may add years to your life. In fact, one study found that just trying to lose weight – even if you don't succeed – can help you live longer. That may be because, in an effort to reduce your weight, you are likely to eat more nutritious foods and practice a healthier lifestyle in other ways, too.

Stop wondering if you're at risk. You may be unsure if the weight you've added over the years is enough to affect your health. Here are some ways to find out.

▶ Compare apples and pears. Look in the mirror and note where your extra weight is located. Fat stored around your waistline is much more dangerous to your health than fat stored on your hips and thighs. In fact, fat around your waist, giving you an apple shape, puts you at higher risk for heart disease than if a few extra pounds have settled in the lower part of your body, giving you a pear-shaped appearance.

▶ Measure your middle. Just how much girth is a problem? Consider your health at risk if you are a woman with a waist measurement of more than 35 inches. If you are a man, 40 inches or more means it's time to reduce. Even with a smaller measurement, you may still be at risk for health problems if your waistline has increased 2 inches or more since you reached maturity.

▶ Check the charts. Use the body mass index (BMI) chart on page 251 to determine the ratio of your weight to your height. This will help you decide if your weight is in a healthy range. A BMI between 19 and 25 is considered healthy. A BMI above 25 generally means you are overweight, and over 30 indicates you are obese, a more serious health concern. This index is based on the assumption that having extra weight means you have more body fat. If, however, you are muscular you may fall into an overweight category but still be healthy. As you get older, waist measurement may be a more accurate indicator of obesity than BMI. Many seniors lose muscle mass as they gain fat. That means it's possible to fall within the healthy weight category when, in fact, you're carrying too much unhealthy fat.

▶ Get expert advice. Not all seniors should go on a diet. Talk to your doctor, especially if you are older than 65 or plan to lose more than 20 pounds. Be sure to discuss the cause of your weight gain, and find out how other health conditions, like diabetes and high blood pressure, come into play.

Be kind to your heart. Carrying extra weight brings extra risks to your heart. People with a BMI of 30 or higher have a risk of dying that's 50 to 100 percent higher than for those with a lower BMI. The main danger is heart disease. Extra weight causes several unhealthy changes to your circulatory system.

▶ Blood vessels become injured. Particularly if you carry lots of weight around your middle, your body may be producing extra C-reactive protein (CRP). Experts say CRP is a sign of inflammation and damaged arteries.

▶ Higher weight means higher blood pressure. If you have big numbers on both counts, losing weight can reduce your risk for serious problems.

▶ Heart failure is more common. Even if other dangerous conditions like high blood pressure and diabetes are factored in, obese people still have a higher risk for heart failure.

▶ Cholesterol levels get out of whack. Obese people tend to have higher levels of dangerous triglycerides and lower levels of HDL or "good" cholesterol.

▶ Strokes are more common.

6 slick tricks to keep off the pounds

It's normal for pounds to creep up as the years go by. But common sense and a healthy plan of attack will help you keep off extra weight.

▶ Drink water every day.

▶ Eat plenty of whole grains, legumes, and fresh fruits and vegetables.

▶ Cut back on sweets, refined carbohydrates, processed foods, and unhealthy fats.

▶ Get at least 30 minutes of moderate exercise every day.

▶ Keep a food diary, writing down everything you eat.

▶ Sit down to eat, concentrate on your food, and push the plate aside when you're full — whether it's empty or not.

Body mass index (BMI) chart

Weight Height	100	110	120	130	140	150	160	170	180	190	200
5'0"	20	21	23	25	27	29	31	33	35	37	39
5'1"	19	21	23	25	26	28	30	32	34	36	38
5'2"	18	20	22	24	26	27	29	31	33	35	37
5'3"	18	19	21	23	25	27	28	30	32	34	35
5'4"	17	19	21	22	24	26	27	29	31	33	34
5'5"	17	18	20	22	23	25	27	28	30	32	33
5'6"	16	18	19	21	23	24	26	27	29	31	32
5'7"	16	17	19	20	22	23	25	27	28	30	31
5'8"	15	17	18	20	21	23	24	26	27	29	30
5'9"	15	16	18	19	21	22	24	25	27	28	30
5'10"	14	16	17	19	20	22	23	24	26	27	29
5'11"	14	15	17	18	20	21	22	24	25	26	28
6'0"	14	15	16	18	19	20	22	23	24	26	27
6'1"	13	15	16	17	18	20	21	22	24	25	26
6'2"	13	14	15	17	18	19	21	22	23	24	26
6'3"	12	14	15	16	17	19	20	21	22	24	25

Lose weight without even trying

Some foods practically force your body to lose weight. Eight to try are whole-grain bread, soup, apples, oranges, broccoli, lentils, brown rice, and Canadian bacon. The secret — they help you feel full while adding fewer calories to your diet.

Fill up on whole grains. Results are in from a study of 27,000 people — eat whole grains if you want to lose weight. Eating more whole-grain foods, especially those made with bran, kept men slimmer over the course of eight years. The more they ate, the less weight they gained. What's more, other research shows choosing whole grains over refined ones actually helps you lose weight.

Whole grains are rich in fiber, and experts think filling up on high-fiber foods helps you eat less throughout the day. They pack fewer calories per ounce than foods made with refined grains, like white flour or white rice, and they satisfy hunger better, to boot. This is the perfect way to lose weight without going hungry.

Choose foods made with bran, and check food labels for whole-grain ingredients, including "whole oats" and "cracked wheat." Consider drinking a glass of orange juice with a psyllium fiber supplement, like Fiberall, stirred in 30 minutes before every meal, and you'll be well on your way to a slimmer you.

Save room for soup. It's the one food you can eat and eat and still lose weight. Soup is a food with low energy density, meaning a single cup contains fewer calories than most other foods. It also takes up a lot of room in your stomach, so it satisfies hunger better. Eating two servings every day of soup helped dieters lose 50 percent more weight than eating other snacks with the same number of calories. The soup-slurpers felt fuller throughout the day, which may have helped them snack less.

Skip the cream-based soups, which are heavy in fat and high in calories. Instead, enjoy those with a vegetable- or chicken-broth base and loaded with high-fiber foods, like brown rice, vegetables, and lentils. Try to eat more fruits and vegetables with high water, fiber, and nutrient content, such as apples or broccoli.

Pile on the protein. The right breakfast – one that includes a little lean protein – could keep you full until lunch. In a Purdue University study, women who added a slice of Canadian bacon to their breakfast felt less hungry for four hours than those who skipped the protein. This nutrient makes your body release the hunger-reducing hormone PYY, so you snack less during the day.

Eat slowly. It does help you eat less. Experts gave two groups of college women the same meal but told one group to eat fast and the other to chew each bite 15 to 20 times. The slow-eaters not only ate 67 fewer calories, they also felt fuller than the fast-eaters for an hour afterward.

Energy densities of 3 popular foods

Low-density foods, like fruits and vegetables, are bulky and filling, without a lot of calories. But high-density foods have a ton of calories jammed into small servings, mainly because they're loaded with fats and sugars.

Food	Calories	Weight of food	Food density
medium apple	71	138 grams	$71 \div 138 = 0.5$ (low energy density)
tuna fish salad (1 cup)	383	205 grams	$383 \div 205 = 1.9$ (medium energy density)
milk chocolate bar	235	44 grams	$235 \div 44 = 5.3$ (high energy density)

Wise up to dangers of popular diet plan

Eat a juicy burger for lunch and a sizzling steak for dinner — and still lose weight. That's the undeniable appeal of high-protein diets.

These popular diets let you load up on meat, cheese, eggs, and other usual dieting outlaws, while severely limiting carbohydrates, such as fruits, vegetables, and bread.

Weight-loss programs like the Atkins Diet or the Zone Diet may help you lose weight in the short term, but they raise some health concerns. In fact, the American Heart Association (AHA) recently issued a warning about high-protein, low-carbohydrate diets. If you want a healthy heart, it's better to cut back on sweets, refined carbohydrates, processed foods, and unhealthy fats and increase whole grains, legumes, and fresh fruits and vegetables in your diet.

Beware of the health dangers. The following possible side effects suggest a high-protein diet is not a safe, long-term solution.

▶ High cholesterol. With all that meat comes a lot of saturated fat, the kind that causes cholesterol buildup in your arteries. You may lose weight but increase your risk for heart disease and stroke. In fact, a 15-year study of women who substituted protein for carbs found those who ate more red meat and dairy products had a higher risk of heart disease.

▶ High blood pressure. When you limit foods like fruits, vegetables, and whole grains, you're eliminating natural ways to lower your blood pressure.

▶ Gout. Foods high in protein are often high in purines, which are converted into uric acid. This can build up and cause gout.

▶ Osteoporosis. Overloading on protein causes your body to get rid of more calcium, leaving your bones weak and brittle.

▶ Cancer. Fewer fruits, vegetables, and whole grains mean fewer cancer-fighting weapons.

▶ Diabetic renal disease. Too much protein can put a strain on your kidneys, making a high-protein diet especially dangerous for people with diabetes.

▶ Vitamin and mineral deficiencies. The lack of healthy foods in your diet means you're not getting all the nutrients you need.

▶ Fatigue and muscle loss. Carbohydrates are your main source of energy. If you cut them out, you can become fatigued after exercising. Get fewer than 100 grams of carbohydrates a day, and your body will resort to burning muscle tissue for energy.

Health issues aside, high-protein diets are generally boring and hard to stick to. You need some variety and excitement in any meal plan to make it work in the long run.

Check out the research. Atkins is a marketing success — more than 45 million books sold and 20 million followers. But while millions of dollars have been spent promoting the low-carb scheme, nutritionists have been investigating the hidden health facts.

A major British medical journal reviewed hundreds of studies on low-carb diets. Three of them, all major randomized trials, have led researchers to conclude:

▶ People trying to lose weight find it harder to stick with low-carb diets than conventional diets.

▶ The long-term safety of low-carb diets can't be guaranteed. Many health professionals are worried about an increase in high cholesterol, low blood sugar, colon cancer, and constipation in people following these diets.

▶ The most solid scientific advice for those who want to lose weight and keep it off is not to radically reduce carbs. It's to cut calories and fat; eat the right combination of foods, like fruits, vegetables, whole grains, and low-fat dairy products; and exercise regularly.

▶ There's evidence that weight lost on low-carb diets doesn't stay off.

The secret to weight loss does not lie with some specific proportion of nutrients or the magic powers of protein. It lies with burning more calories than you take in. In fact, experts say it's the reduced calories, not the additional protein, that helps you lose weight on high-protein diets.

Your body does need protein to function properly. Recent studies suggest older people may need slightly more — but don't go overboard. Your best bet is to eat a balanced diet. The AHA recommends getting about 55 percent of each day's calories from carbohydrates, 20 to 35 percent from fat, and just 15 percent from protein. If you decide you want to try a high-protein diet, make sure you talk to your doctor first.

Get a grip on carb counting

Low-carb eating means getting 30 grams or less of carbohydrates per day. That's about 10 grams per meal. Here's a sampling of what 10 grams — give or take a gram — look like:

▸ about 3/4 cup of low-fat milk

▸ 8 ounces whole-milk plain yogurt

▸ 1/4 cup low-fat vanilla ice cream

▸ a little less than 1/2 cup of cooked oatmeal

▸ about 1/4 cup cooked spaghetti

▸ one extra-thin slice of bread

▸ one tablespoon cough syrup

▸ one small banana

▸ one kiwi fruit

▸ two medium carrots

▸ 1/5 baked potato

▸ 1/4 cup prune juice

▸ 1/3 cup Coke

Make friends with healthy fats

Fat is not your enemy — excess consumption of it is. In fact, without some fat in your diet, your body wouldn't be able to make nerve cells or hormones or absorb the fat-soluble vitamins — A, D, E, and K.

Eat a little fat to feel full. Some researchers believe eating small amounts of fat can actually keep people from overindulging on total calories. Ohio State University nutrition scientist John Allred points out that dietary fat causes your body to produce a hormone that tells your intestines to slow down the emptying process.

This could explain why adding a little peanut butter to your rice cake may satisfy your hunger longer and prevent you from wolfing down the whole bag of rice cakes later.

Certain fats, like olive oil and the omega-3 fatty acids found in cold-water fish, like salmon, may help prevent heart disease. And most people say a little fat simply makes food taste, look, and smell more appetizing.

Know your limits. The U.S. Department of Health and Human Services recommends that you limit the fat in your diet to 20 to 35 percent or less of total calories.

One way to figure this is to make sure all the food you eat meets this guideline. No food you choose to eat should have more than 3 grams of fat for every 100 calories. If you decide to splurge on a favorite high-fat food, you can compensate by limiting your fat calories for the rest of the day or week.

Be picky. The easiest rule to remember is to stay away from saturated fats, such as those in cheese, butter, whole milk, and meat — as well as a few vegetable fats, like coconut oil, palm oil, and hydrogenated vegetable shortenings. During the hydrogenation process, fats are changed to trans fatty acids, which have much the same effect on your body as saturated fats. Less than 10 percent of your calories should come from saturated fats.

You should also limit the polyunsaturated fats you eat to less than 10 percent of your calories. Common sources are safflower oil, soybean oil, and sunflower oil. Monounsaturated fats are the good guys. Olive oil and canola oil are high in monosaturated fats.

Pass the prune purée, please. Many people find that the worst part of weight loss is cutting back on favorite foods or feeling guilty when they do indulge a little. Here's where a little prune purée can come in handy. Use it as the butter, shortening, or oil substitute in your favorite brownie, cake, cookie, or bread recipe.

One cup of prune purée has 407 calories and 1 gram of fat, while one cup of butter has 1,600 calories and 182 grams of fat, and one cup of oil has 1,944 calories and 218 grams of fat. Using prune purée, you save a bundle in fat and calories while indulging your sweet tooth.

To make enough prune purée for several recipes, mix one pound of dried, pitted prunes with one cup of hot water and purée in a food processor. Keep your purée refrigerated in a covered jar.

Giggle away your flab

The next time you're deciding what to watch on television, opt for a comedy. You burn 20 percent more calories when you're laughing. Having a good hoot for 15 minutes burns up to 40 calories, enough for a piece of chocolate. Laugh like that every day for a year, and you could lose 4.4 pounds — it's no joke.

---

7 secrets for a slimmer you

Controlling your weight is not just about what you eat and how much you exercise. It's true — much of the blame for obesity goes to poor eating habits. But that's not the whole story. Without making a few lifestyle changes, you'll always have a hard time maintaining a healthy weight. Here are some tips to help you.

Get your beauty rest. Don't be tempted to get by on less sleep. Achieving a flat tummy may be related to how much sleep you enjoy on a regular basis. Women who sleep only five or six hours a night gain more weight than those who get seven hours of sleep a night, according to the Nurses' Health Study. Another study found that two key hormones that regulate appetite get out of whack when you don't get enough sleep. Leptin, which tells your body you've eaten enough, decreases, and ghrelin, which stimulates your appetite, increases.

Don't overdo it at the table. Researchers at Cornell University discovered something interesting while hosting an ice cream social. When people serve themselves, they tend to put more food on their plates if the plates and serving utensils are large. Think small and cut back on the size of your helpings by using smaller plates, bowls, and serving utensils. Don't fall for the fast food "supersize" craze when you eat out.

Take a break from television. Your risk for obesity increases 23 percent for every two hours a day you spend in front of your TV. Americans now burn 111 less calories a day than in years past, and that adds up to 11 pounds a year. When you're sitting around watching TV, not only does your metabolism slow, you might be tempted by clever advertisers to reach for high-sugar, high-fat snacks – and empty calories.

Share your time with others. Retirees who joined a program to help mentor and tutor children in local elementary schools more than doubled their physical activity, a Johns Hopkins University survey shows. Not only did the volunteers get off the couch and away from the TV, they had more energy for daily activities like household chores and gardening.

Find strength in numbers. You can lose more weight by joining an organized weight-loss group than trying to go it alone, says a study funded by the U.S. Department of Agriculture. Women dieting on their own have higher stress levels, and that leads to less success overall. A group also gives you support and nutritional information you won't get by yourself.

Deal with feelings without food. When you eat to cope with anger, depression, or stress, you're loading up on food that makes you fat. Find something else to help you deal with your emotions – go for a walk, take a relaxing bath, or play a game.

Stay on schedule. Eating three meals a day and a healthful snack or two keeps your blood sugar stable and your hunger pangs under control. In addition, missing a meal can encourage you to overeat at the next meal. Overeating stretches your stomach, which continues to signal hunger until it gets back to normal size.

Dangerous weight-loss shortcut

Don't be tempted to use diuretics, or water pills, to lose weight. They can disturb your body's electrolyte balance and put you at risk of a heart attack. They're especially dangerous when combined with a low-protein diet, which can starve your heart muscle and disturb heart rhythms. Using water pills when taking other medicines is also risky business.

"People taking diuretics are particularly vulnerable to dehydration," says cardiologist Dr. David Calhoun, director of the University of Alabama Birmingham Hypertension Clinic. "The combination of depleted fluid volume and medication," he warns, "can lead to problems such as dangerously low blood pressure, particularly for older patients who are sensitive to becoming dehydrated."

If you take medications, Calhoun says, be sure to drink at least the recommended six glasses of water each day — more when you exercise or spend time in the sun.

Diet pills you should know about

Diet pills and potions are big business these days. Do they work? Sometimes — but only when you adopt some lifestyle changes, like cutting calories and exercising more. What they won't do is magically melt pounds away while you sit on your couch and eat whatever you want.

Your doctor may prescribe one of several drugs to either curb your appetite or prevent your body from absorbing some of the fat you eat if you are obese. Most of these weight-loss drugs are approved for short-term use, and they all have unpleasant side effects. Some are mild, like headaches or stomach cramps, but others are serious, like high blood pressure.

Here's something else to consider — most weight-loss drugs lose their effectiveness over time, and some can become addictive or trigger depression. These drugs don't work the same for everyone, so the exact dosage and results vary. Currently, three types of weight-loss drugs are available.

Fat absorption inhibitors. These drugs reduce your body's absorption of some of the fat you eat. They come with unpleasant side effects, like gas and diarrhea, and they interfere with absorption of the fat-soluble vitamins A, D, and E and other important nutrients. The only fat absorption inhibitor approved by the U.S. Food and Drug Administration (FDA) is orlistat (Xenical). It's also available in a weaker, over-the-counter version called Alli.

Metabolism boosters. These compounds are part of a host of unregulated diet remedies, which also include appetite suppressants not approved by the FDA. This approach to weight loss, known as thermogenic therapy, suggests that certain natural compounds, like chromium and pyruvate, encourage your liver to increase energy in your cells and stimulate metabolism. They all have numerous side effects — many of them serious.

Appetite suppressants. These include the many herbs, drugs, and supplements sold to either curb your appetite or make you feel full. Phentermine — the "phen" part of the discontinued diet drug Fen-phen — is the most common prescription appetite suppressant. Brand names, including Adipex and Ionamin, can cost two or more times as much as generic phentermine. Fen-phen was banned several years ago because fenfluramine, the "fen" ingredient, was linked to heart valve problems. Phentermine is not associated with heart problems. Other prescription appetite suppressants include sibutramine (Meridia) and diethylpropion (Tenuate). The appetite suppressant industry is a graveyard, literally in some cases, of failed claims. While the jury may still be out on the new arrivals, it's wise not to become a guinea pig for the latest pill when there are healthy alternatives.

Contrave, a combination of two older drugs, bupropion and naltrexone, might substantially lower blood sugar, control cholesterol levels, and promote weight loss. Studies show this "wonder pill" combo may control your appetite so you can eat less and lose weight. Much of the weight people lose is fat in the abdomen, where it's the most dangerous. Contrave also seems to improve risk factors like high triglycerides, cholesterol, and insulin resistance. More studies are being done to see how Contrave can help people with type 2 diabetes.

Experts say the best – and safest – way to lose weight and keep it off is to eat less and exercise more. Over-the-counter pills and so-called natural remedies are expensive, and they can cause dangerous side effects. Besides that, their reactions with other drugs are unknown.

Straight talk about weight-loss scams

You want to lose weight, and you want to lose it now. So those advertisements for diets, pills, body wraps, patches, and creams really catch your attention. It's hard to resist their promises – no matter how unbelievable they may sound. Fantastic guarantees, however, should be your first clue that the claims may not be trustworthy. If the quick fix seems too easy, like swallowing a calorie blocker or a fat magnet pill before you eat, it is too good to be true.

Also, don't be fooled by a name that seems reliable, like the Mayo Clinic Diet, for example. The truth is, the Mayo Clinic has never given its backing to a grapefruit diet, an egg diet, or any of the many other quick weight-loss plans that use its name.

Quick-fix diets waste your money and cause you to delay getting started on a nutritious eating plan. If you do lose weight on one of these programs, you are likely to gain it back quickly. Worse still are diet pills, which can be a deadly mistake. Unfortunately, almost everybody is tempted to try them when they want to get rid of weight fast.

Remember the "wonder drug" fen-phen? It was taken off the market because it caused heart damage. And phenylpropanolamine (PPA), an ingredient in some diet pills now banned, made blood pressure shoot dangerously high. In 2004 the U.S. Food and Drug Administration (FDA) banned all products containing ephedra, or ma huang. There's evidence it causes heart attacks, strokes, and seizures.

It seems as fast as one dangerous diet pill is taken off the market, an untested substitute is there to take its place. Bitter orange, or *Citrus aurantium*, is a current favorite. It's harmless in small amounts as a flavoring for food, but it contains a compound, synephrine, that works in much the same way as ephedra.

Experts believe the amounts of bitter orange found in over-the-counter supplements can raise your blood pressure and cause heart problems, especially if you take them in combination with other stimulants, like caffeine. It can also interact with certain prescription medications.

But here's the good news. A healthy eating and lifestyle program will help you lose weight safely and keep it off for the rest of your life.

Super strategies for successful weight control

Every year, losing weight ranks as the most common New Year's resolution. Then, 365 days older and a few pounds heavier, people make the same resolution again. But that extra weight puts you at extra risk for health problems, including diabetes, heart disease, high blood pressure, and certain forms of cancer. So ring in the next new year the right way – with a smart, healthy approach to weight control.

Many people want to lose a few pounds. Unfortunately, not everyone goes about it in a healthy way. Dieting can actually cause weight gain and lead to serious illness of the mind and body. This is especially true if you fall into the pattern of yo-yo dieting – losing weight, gaining it back, losing again, gaining it back again.

Beware of quick-fix promises, "miracle" products, and fad diets. Pills, body wraps, patches, and creams may tempt you, but there is really no easy way to lose weight. If it sounds too good to be true, it probably is. Diet pills can be worse than ineffective – they can be dangerous. Many contain untested and potentially harmful ingredients.

Restrictive diets – like the high-protein, low-carbohydrate Atkins Diet – may help you lose weight, but they often do not provide adequate nutrition. For instance, you may not get enough fruits, vegetables, or whole grains. The long-term effects of such diets, which are high in saturated fats, remain unknown. Besides that, it's hard to stick to such a limited diet, so you are more likely to give up and gain the weight back.

Rather than rely on gimmicks, get-slim-quick schemes, and the latest "in" diet, consider these effective and safe weight-control strategies. The key is to follow a healthy eating plan for life – as opposed to crash dieting a few weeks before the next class reunion. Here are six ways to lose weight that actually work.

▶ Eat only what you can burn. That's the secret to weight control. No specific foods are forbidden. Just remember if you eat that slice of cheesecake, you need to burn off those calories. Your body generally burns 1,800 to 2,000 calories per day.

▶ Control your portions. Restaurant portions have steadily grown – and so have Americans' waistlines. When you dine out, remember you don't have to clean your plate. At home, pay attention to a food's suggested serving size. You'd be surprised how many servings you might be eating at one time. If necessary, use a smaller plate to trick yourself into eating smaller portions.

▶ Aim for more plant than animal foods. Think of meat as the side dish and vegetables as the entree. Plant-based foods should cover at least two-thirds of your plate. Eat half your usual portion of meat and have two veggies instead of one.

▸ Exercise regularly. Eating less plus moving more equals subtracted pounds. Aim for one hour a day of moderate exercise. Your activity can be as simple as going for a walk.

▸ Keep a food diary. Take note of what you eat and how you feel.

▸ Set realistic goals. Expect to lose about 10 percent of your weight. Slow and steady wins the race. When you reach small goals, reward yourself — but not with food.

Burn extra calories while you play	
Fitness activity	**Calories burned ***
tennis (singles)	275
bicycling (no hills)	221
racquetball	221
aerobics	203
badminton (singles)	198
yoga	180
tennis (doubles)	171
ballroom dancing	153
water aerobics	144
swing dancing	135
table tennis	135
tai chi	135
golfing (no cart)	131
strolling	104

* The number of calories a 150-pound person would burn for 30 minutes of activity.

3 great reasons to eat more fiber

If dietary fiber didn't already exist, some weight-loss genius would be working overtime in the laboratory trying to invent it.

This natural substance, found in fruits, vegetables, and whole grains, not only helps prevent disease, lower cholesterol, and keep you regular — it also helps you lose weight. Read on to discover how fiber zaps away pounds.

Blocks calories. Good news — you can eat as much fiber as your body can handle and add absolutely no calories to your diet. What's more, your body needs fiber to function at its peak.

Many of fiber's calories don't count because insoluble fiber can't be digested. It just passes through your system, taking waste with it. Fiber can also block the absorption of some of the fat and protein you eat. One study found that people who ate 48 grams of fiber a day absorbed 8 percent fewer calories than those who got a daily dose of 20 grams of fiber.

Just boosting your fiber intake — without changing the number of calories you eat — could mean losing a couple of pounds a month. But make sure to add fiber to your diet gradually. Too much too fast can cause uncomfortable gas and bloating.

Fills you up. Like Doug Henning or David Copperfield, fiber is a skilled illusionist. Even though it isn't digested, it still fills you up. High-fiber foods trick your stomach into feeling full with fewer calories than you would normally eat. You also stay full longer, meaning you won't feel the urge to snack between meals.

Drink plenty of water as you add more fiber to your diet. Fiber absorbs water and swells, giving you that satisfied, full feeling. The main thing is, fiber works. A recent review of popular diet plans found that people eating a low-fat, high-fiber diet lost more than three times as much weight as people on a low-fat diet alone.

Clobbers bad cholesterol. Fiber has another secret benefit. It helps lower bad LDL cholesterol, while keeping your good HDL cholesterol steady. So your heart, as well as your mirror, will thank you.

Plan for success

They say failing to plan is planning to fail. That certainly applies to weight control. You have many options, including the Pritikin Plan. The basic elements of this program, which has been around since the 1970s, include a diet low in fat, calories, and salt — as well as making time for moderate exercise.

Keep in mind that an extremely low-fat diet — one that limits fat to 10 percent of your total calories — may not be ideal for heart health. While this type of diet will lower bad LDL cholesterol, it also reduces your helpful HDL cholesterol and may raise triglycerides.

With such little fat allowed, you may not get enough healthy fats, like omega-3 fatty acids. Your body may also have trouble absorbing important fat-soluble vitamins, such as vitamins A, E, D, and K. Following a very low-fat diet also means radically changing your eating habits. This makes it tough to stick to, especially when dining out. A less-restrictive diet, with a more moderate fat intake, may be a more realistic option. For more information, call the Pritikin Longevity Center at 800-327-4914, or check the Web site at *www.pritikin.com*.

High-fiber recipes for healthy eating

Try these high-fiber recipes, loaded with this natural appetite suppressant. Fiber blocks the absorption of fat, fills you up so you don't overeat, and helps you take off extra pounds. Eureka! What a magnificent invention.

Zucchini lasagna

1/2 pound lasagna noodles, cooked in unsalted water

2 1/2 cups no-salt-added tomato sauce

1 1/2 cups raw zucchini, sliced

2 teaspoons basil, dried

1/4 cup onion, chopped

1/8 teaspoon black pepper

3/4 cup part-skim mozzarella cheese, grated

1 1/2 cups fat-free cottage cheese

1/4 cup Parmesan cheese, grated

2 teaspoons oregano, dried

1 clove garlic

1. Preheat oven to 350 degrees Fahrenheit. Lightly spray 9- by 13-inch baking dish with canola oil spray.

2. In small bowl, combine 1/8 cup mozzarella and 1 tablespoon Parmesan cheese. Set aside.

3. In medium bowl, combine remaining mozzarella and Parmesan cheese with all of the cottage cheese. Mix well and set aside.

4. Combine tomato sauce with remaining ingredients. Spread thin layer of tomato sauce in bottom of baking dish. Add a third of noodles in single layer. Spread half of cottage cheese mixture on top. Add layer of zucchini.

5. Repeat layering. Add thin coating of sauce. Top with noodles, sauce, and reserved cheese mixture. Cover with aluminum foil.

6. Bake for 30 to 40 minutes. Cool for about 15 minutes. Cut into 6 portions.

Yield: 6 servings

Each serving provides:
total fat: 5 grams (g)
cholesterol: 11 milligrams (mg)
total fiber: 5 g
carbohydrates: 41 g

Serving size: 1 piece

calories: 276
saturated fat: 2 g
sodium: 380 mg
protein: 19 g
potassium: 561 mg

Recipe courtesy of U.S. Department of Health and Human Services, National Institutes of Health.

Black skillet beef with greens and red potatoes

1 pound top round beef	1 tablespoon paprika
1 1/2 teaspoons oregano	1/2 teaspoon chili powder
1/4 teaspoon garlic powder	1/4 teaspoon black pepper
1/8 teaspoon red pepper	1/8 teaspoon dry mustard
8 red-skinned potatoes, halved	3 cups onion, finely chopped
2 cups beef broth	2 large cloves of garlic, minced
2 large carrots, peeled, cut into very thin, 2 1/2-inch strips	2 bunches (1/2 pound) mustard greens, kale, or turnip greens, stems removed, coarsely torn

canola oil spray, as needed

1. Partially freeze beef. Thinly slice across grain into long strips 1/8 inch thick and 3 inches wide.

2. Combine paprika, oregano, chili powder, garlic powder, black pepper, red pepper, and dry mustard. Coat strips of meat with spice mixture.

3. Spray large, heavy skillet with canola oil spray. Preheat pan over high heat. Add meat and cook for 5 minutes, stirring often. Then add potatoes, onion, broth, and garlic, and cook covered over medium heat for 20 minutes. Stir in carrots, lay greens over top, and cook covered until carrots are tender, about 15 minutes.

4. Serve in large serving bowl with crusty bread for dunking.

Yield: 6 servings

Serving size: 7 oz

Each serving provides:
total fat: 5 grams (g)
cholesterol: 64 milligrams (mg)
total fiber: 8 g
carbohydrates: 45 g

calories: 340
saturated fat: 2 g
sodium: 109 mg
protein: 30 g
potassium: 1,278 mg

Recipe courtesy of U.S. Department of Health and Human Services, National Institutes of Health.

New Orleans red beans

1 pound dry red beans

2 quarts water

1 1/2 cups onion, chopped

1 cup celery, chopped

4 bay leaves

1 cup green peppers, chopped

3 tablespoons garlic, chopped

3 tablespoons parsley, chopped

2 teaspoons dried thyme, crushed

1 teaspoon salt

1 teaspoon black pepper

1. Pick through beans to remove bad ones. Rinse beans thoroughly.

2. In large pot, combine beans, water, onion, celery, and bay leaves. Bring to boil. Reduce heat, cover, and cook over low heat for about 1 1/2 hours or until beans are tender. Stir. Mash beans against side of pan.

3. Add green pepper, garlic, parsley, thyme, salt, and black pepper. Cook uncovered over low heat until creamy, about 30 minutes. Remove bay leaves.

4. Serve with hot cooked brown rice, if desired.

Yield: 8 servings

Serving size: 1 1/4 cups

Each serving provides:

calories: 171

total fat: less than 1 gram (g)

saturated fat: less than 1 g

cholesterol: 0 milligrams (mg)

sodium: 285 mg

total fiber: 7 g

protein: 10 g

carbohydrates: 32 g

potassium: 665 mg

Recipe courtesy of U.S. Department of Health and Human Services, National Institutes of Health.

Sunshine rice

1 1/2 tablespoons canola oil

1 1/2 cups onion, finely chopped

1 cup water

2 tablespoons lemon juice

1/4 cup slivered almonds

1 1/4 cups celery, finely chopped, with leaves

1 cup long-grain white rice, uncooked

1/2 cup orange juice

dash hot sauce

1. Heat oil in medium saucepan. Add celery and onions and sauté until tender (about 10 minutes).

2. Add water, juices, and hot sauce. Bring to boil. Stir in rice and bring back to boil. Let stand covered until rice is tender and liquid is absorbed.

3. Stir in almonds. Serve immediately.

Yield: 4 servings

Each serving provides:
total fat: 6 grams (g)
cholesterol: 0 milligrams (mg)
total fiber: 5 g
carbohydrates: 50 g

Serving size: 1/3 cup

calories: 276
saturated fat: 1 g
sodium: 52 mg
protein: 7 g
potassium: 406 mg

Recipe courtesy of U.S. Department of Health and Human Services, National Institutes of Health.

Winter crisp

For filling:

1/2 cup sugar	3 tablespoons all-purpose flour
1 teaspoon lemon peel, grated	3/4 teaspoon lemon juice
5 cups apples, unpeeled, sliced	1 cup cranberries

For topping:

2/3 cup rolled oats	1/3 cup brown sugar, packed
1/4 cup whole-wheat flour	2 teaspoons ground cinnamon
1 tablespoon soft margarine, melted	

1. Prepare filling by combining sugar, flour, and lemon peel in medium bowl. Mix well. Add lemon juice, apples, and cranberries. Stir to mix. Spoon into 6-cup baking dish.

2. Prepare topping by combining oats, brown sugar, flour, and cinnamon in small bowl. Add melted margarine. Stir to mix.

3. Sprinkle topping over filling. Bake in 375-degree Fahrenheit oven for approximately 40 to 50 minutes or until filling is bubbly and top is brown. Serve warm or at room temperature.

Yield: 6 servings   **Serving size: 1 3/4″ by 2″**

Each serving provides:	
total fat: 2 grams (g)	calories: 252
cholesterol: 0 milligrams (mg)	saturated fat: less than 1 g
total fiber: 5 g	sodium: 29 mg
carbohydrates: 58 g	protein: 3 g
	potassium: 221 mg

Recipe courtesy of U.S. Department of Health and Human Services, National Institutes of Health.

7 ways fiber helps you win at losing

You've tried the hot dog diet, the banana diet, and the grapefruit diet. You've gone through diet pills, sweat suits, and supplements. Your home is littered with exercise equipment and videos that promised to help you lose those extra pounds. But despite your best efforts, you can't seem to lose weight. What are you doing wrong?

Chances are, you're not eating enough fiber. Studies show obesity rates are tied to the amount of fiber people eat. In places like Kenya and Uganda, where they eat as much as 60 to 80 grams of fiber daily, less than 15 percent of the population is overweight. But the measly 15 grams a day eaten in more modern societies, like the United States, have contributed to the obesity of nearly 60 percent of adults.

If you're one of them, you'll need to change your diet to include more fruits and vegetables because most fiber comes from plants. You'll find it in whole-grain foods, legumes, leafy vegetables, fruits, nuts, root vegetables and their skins, and bran flakes. Besides allowing you more food on your plate, this important diet aid works on several levels to keep you trim.

Offers more food per calorie. One of the best things about fiber is that some of its calories don't count. That's because much of dietary fiber can't be digested. But fiber still fills you up. Experts say eating a diet high in fiber can trick your stomach into feeling full with fewer calories than you would normally eat.

Prolongs your meal. Most people would agree that the pleasure of food lies in the eating. A high-fiber diet requires lots of chewing and swallowing, and it can take a good while to finish a meal. Unlike many diets that limit food, you won't have to give up the joy of eating when you add fiber to your diet. It might actually take you longer than usual to polish off a lower-calorie meal.

Bulks up in your stomach. Ever finish a small meal while dieting and still feel hunger pangs? That won't happen if you eat more fiber. Water-soluble fiber absorbs water from your stomach and forms a kind of gel that swells up. Nerve receptors in your stomach signal your brain that your stomach is full, and you no longer need to eat. By filling up on fiber, you can go about your business without constantly feeling hungry.

Keeps you satisfied longer. But that's not all fiber can do. The thick gel it forms slows down the movement of food out of your stomach, so you end up processing your food more slowly. Instead of a high-calorie blast of energy that is quickly followed by tiredness and hunger, your energy supply is spread out over time.

Stabilizes blood sugar. Experts say this process affects your blood sugar in a healthy way. When you eat dried beans, barley, whole wheat, or pumpernickel bread, these foods slowly release their sugars for energy. Instead of your body getting surges of sugar from food, it gets its energy in steady amounts, which helps control insulin levels. In addition, a high-fiber meal can affect your blood sugar's response to the next meal you eat, keeping your blood sugar more stable throughout the day.

Boosts your hormones. You may not know it, but you have hormones working in your gastrointestinal tract. One in particular, called GLP-1, slows down the digestion process and gives you a sense of fullness. It can also help you lose weight. Studies on animals showed that eating fermentable fiber — the kind in fruits and vegetables — boosted their levels of GLP-1.

Blocks some calories. Dietary fiber can block the absorption of some of the fat and protein you eat. If you're overweight, that could be a good thing. One study showed that a group of people fed a diet containing only 20 grams of fiber a day absorbed 8 percent more calories than a group given 48 grams of fiber a day. For a typical 2,500-calorie diet, that's a difference of about 200 calories a day.

Just changing your fiber intake — without altering the number of calories you eat — could mean losing a couple of pounds a month. But be careful to add fiber to your diet slowly. Too much too soon can cause uncomfortable gas and bloating.

Block cravings with feel-good oats

Enjoy the hearty goodness of oats, and you might not crave sweets, bread, and pasta. That's because those cravings can mean your brain has low levels of serotonin, a chemical that affects sensations and mood.

Your brain can make serotonin from tryptophan, an essential amino acid found in protein-rich foods. Just eating foods like turkey, dairy products, and nuts can get tryptophan into your blood. But you need carbohydrates to move tryptophan into your brain. All carbohydrates stimulate this serotonin production, but researchers at the University of South Alabama found that complex carbs, like oats, oatmeal, beans, and whole grains, also have a long-lasting mood-lifting effect. These delicious foods can improve your mood and stop you from overeating.

But that's not all. The soluble fiber beta glucan gives oats and oat products many other health benefits, including helping to lower your cholesterol.

4 ways to shake off stress and lose weight

Do you stress out because of your weight? Or do you gain weight because of your stress? Turns out both may be true. Stress can have a tremendous effect on your diet, and vice versa. By counting every calorie and obsessing over your food, you could sabotage your weight-loss efforts. Learn how to protect yourself from excess weight caused by stress.

Loosen up. Simply trying to stick to your diet can be stressful. A recent study showed that women on a restricted diet were under more stress. They had more cortisol, a stress hormone, in their bodies than women who didn't limit what they ate. High levels of cortisol can lead to weak, brittle bones, making such constant stress dangerous.

Instead of counting calories and fat grams, adopt a generally healthy diet featuring plenty of fruits, vegetables, and whole grains. You'll lose weight without the stress.

Do something fun. Studies show stress may add to the fat around your middle. Abdominal fat raises your risk for health problems, including heart disease and diabetes. The danger remains even if the rest of your body is lean. In one study of 59 women 30 to 46 years old, the thin women with potbellies seemed more vulnerable to stress than the heavier women.

A great way to cope with stress — and shed some fat — is to exercise regularly. Other good stress-busters include getting a massage, listening to music, taking deep breaths, gardening, laughing, and talking about your troubles with a friend.

Switch snacks. People who eat to cope with stress usually don't make the best food choices. They reach for comfort foods like pizza, sausage, hamburgers, and chocolate — and they also drink more alcohol. Single, divorced, and unemployed men often fall into this trap, as do women who feel they don't get enough emotional support. If stress gives you the urge to snack, try one of the stress-busting techniques mentioned earlier instead. If you absolutely need a snack, reach for an apple or some celery sticks instead of cookies.

Turn off the news. Many people feel constantly stressed and uneasy because of negative news headlines or the dangers they perceive in modern life. Your body responds to this long-term stress by creating fat stores for energy and breaking down muscles to help fight infection.

According to University of Georgia nutrition expert Carolyn Berdanier, eating slightly more polyunsaturated fat and protein can help your body cope with long-term stress. The fat lets your body know it has some energy available, and the protein helps keep your muscles intact. Exercise helps, too.

Whether you modify your diet, your approach to stress, or both, you should be pleasantly surprised the next time you step on the scale.

Beware of common dieting hazard

If you're considering a quick detox diet, think again. Bad things happen to your body when you fast.

▶ The dramatic weight you lose at first is just water.

▶ Soon you're burning fat — but also muscle.

▶ Substances called ketones collect in your body, and your mineral levels drop. Among other things, this could cause severe heart problems.

▶ Your metabolism slows — you burn less fat — and other body processes slow or stop completely.

When you stop fasting, it's likely you will gain weight back quickly — and most of it will come back as fat and water. A long fast can also permanently damage your heart and weaken your immune system.

Don't endanger your health just to lose a few pounds. If you must, fast for no more than 24 hours and drink plenty of water to stay hydrated.

Dieting dozen gets the job done

Are you ready to lose weight, pamper your heart, and feel as energetic as you did 20 years ago? You can't go wrong with these 12 tips for success. They may be the last weight-loss advice you'll ever need. These easy-to-follow tips are based on solid scientific research and sound advice from doctors and nutrition experts.

Begin with a commitment to good health. This chapter contains good advice on what to eat and what to avoid. Make those changes a part of your routine for at least a month. This will lay a strong foundation for lasting weight control.

Prepare yourself mentally. Losing weight permanently and safely is a life-changing concept. Think about the good reasons for wanting to lose weight – better health, more energy, improved appearance. Be sure it's your idea, not someone else's.

Build a support network. Let family and friends know your intention. Spend time with those who encourage you, and avoid those who would throw cold water on your plans.

Set realistic goals. For most, a goal of 1 pound per week – 20 pounds in 20 weeks – is ideal. This may seem like a modest goal, but it's best over the long term. Losing weight slowly but steadily means the weight is more likely to stay off. Certain health problems, like gallstones, can develop if you lose weight too fast. Two pounds per week is the absolute most you should consider losing unless, for health reasons, your doctor supervises you on a quicker plan.

Make a meal plan. Base your daily menus on the number of calories you'll need each day. Choose nutrient-dense foods, as opposed to those with empty calories, and remember to get the recommended number of servings from each food group. As you plan your own meals, be aware of calorie density, too. Carbohydrates and proteins have about four calories per gram, while fat has nine calories – more than twice as many – per gram. So you can fill up on bulky grains and vegetables, for example, and get far fewer calories than from the same amount of fatty meats and desserts. Spread your calories throughout the day. Munching more often on smaller meals will help you lose weight without feeling hungry.

Measure your portions. The actual amounts of food you eat are often different from – and larger than – standard serving sizes. Check yourself by using measuring cups and spoons to determine the size of your portions, at least until you learn to "eyeball" what a serving really is. This will help you more accurately calculate the calories you are actually eating. It will also help show if you are getting all the recommended servings of the different food groups. Read labels on prepared foods for serving sizes.

Don't skip meals. If you want to lose weight fast, your first thought may be to cut out a few meals. But hunger pangs can send you searching desperately for something – anything – to eat.

Keeping to a regular schedule is the best way to assure you won't get hungry. Above all, don't forget to eat breakfast. Nutritionists say it can play a major role in the long-term success of your weight-loss plan.

Determine your eating weaknesses. Everybody has them — those foods you just can't resist. The best way to manage those cravings is to allow small indulgences from time to time. Of course, it's best if your favorite treat also has some health benefit. Although an ounce of dark chocolate, for example, has about 150 calories, it may be good for your heart. If cookies are your weakness, consider those that are fruit-filled, like Fig Newtons. They provide lots of fiber and antioxidant nutrients. If torn between a sweet beverage and a dessert, go for the solid. In one study, people who ate a sweet snack were less hungry and ate less at the next meal than those who drank a sugary drink with the same number of calories.

Take a supplement. Although foods are your best source of nutrients, when you lower your calories, it's a good idea to back up even the most nutritious diet with a daily multiple vitamin and mineral supplement.

Weigh in weekly. Slow but steady weight loss can seem discouraging on a daily basis. Because your weight can change slightly as your body holds and loses water during the day, a weekly reading will be more accurate.

Reward yourself. You'll keep your enthusiasm high if you celebrate small successes. Treat yourself to a massage, go to a movie, or spend time with friends in an activity — like hiking or bowling — that doesn't include food. You can also reward yourself by giving away your old clothes and buying new, smaller ones.

Rest at your new level. Maintain your new weight for a few months, enjoying your success, before you decide if you need to lose any more. If you find you are ready to drop a few more pounds, go back and set a new goal.

Grapefruit battles the bulge

Before you eat a heavy meal, try eating half a grapefruit. Then the fat you eat won't do as much harm. It's true — the old-fashioned "grapefruit diet" may be just a fad, but including this tangy fruit in your weight-loss plan really works. Research shows that over-weight people who ate half a grapefruit before each meal lost an average of 3.6 pounds in a 12-week study.

People in other test groups tried drinking grapefruit juice and taking capsules of dried grapefruit. These groups lost some weight, but not as much as the fruit eaters. Along with grape-fruit's benefits on weight and insulin control, experts say naringin, a flavonoid in grapefruit, slows absorption of fats and carbohydrates in your intestines.

But if you take prescription drugs, check the drug information leaflets or ask your doctor or pharmacist about consuming grapefruit or its juice. Some drugs, like certain calcium-channel blockers and statins, interact with grapefruit juice and may build up to dangerous blood levels.

Old world secret for a long life

People in Mediterranean countries like Greece live longer and suf-fer fewer diseases than people from anywhere else on earth. Their cholesterol may not be that much lower, but fewer die from heart disease or suffer from other chronic illnesses.

Their long, healthy lives have made them famous and given doctors a reason to celebrate. You can share in that good health. Experts have devised an amazing Mediterranean food pyramid based on the tradi-tional eating habits of people in this part of the world. Studies show it seems to protect you from heart disease and certain kinds of cancer.

A recent study shows you may slash your risk of Alzheimer's dis-ease on the Mediterranean eating plan. Researchers followed more than 2,000 older people in New York City, tracking what they ate and whether they showed signs of the disease. Those who most closely adhered to the Mediterranean diet were less likely to develop Alzheimer's disease — up to 40 percent less during the four-year study.

In addition, a Mediterranean eating plan may help you lose weight. Some researchers have found it works better than low-fat diets over the long haul, possibly because it's easier to follow. With the Mediterranean diet, you don't have to make any drastic diet changes, like cutting out all fat or carbohydrates. You can still eat pasta, cheese, and red meat. The key lies in moderation and in eating plenty of whole, unprocessed foods.

The traditional Greek diet is full of fibrous fruits and vegetables, unrefined carbohydrates from whole grains and legumes, and heart-healthy antioxidants, like resveratrol from grapes and red wine, as well as monounsaturated fats and some omega-3 fatty acids from olive oil. At the same time, Greeks tend to get less saturated fat from animal foods.

The result is an eating plan proven to lower LDL cholesterol and ward off heart disease. Rather than animal foods, plants make up the main part of Mediterranean meals. A plate heavy with fresh fruits, legumes, simple vegetables, and whole-grain pastas and breads sits in the middle of this healthy table. Some experts believe the nutrients in these whole plant foods — fiber, antioxidants, and unrefined carbohydrates — provide the protective effects of the Mediterranean diet. Here's how to snag the same benefits.

Eat your veggies — and your fruits. Put a variety of fruits and vegetables at the top of your grocery list, and eat between seven and 10 servings of them each day. Avoid using heavy cream and butter sauces on your produce. Opt instead for steaming or stir-frying vegetables in olive oil.

Say hello to whole grains. Add whole-grain breads, cereals, and other unrefined grains, like brown rice, couscous, bulgur, or polenta for a hefty dose of fiber. Avoid refined grains such as white bread, biscuits, and baked goods.

Belly up to the beans. Make legumes and tree nuts a regular part of your day. Soybeans, peas, lentils, and other beans are top-notch legumes, while walnuts, almonds, and pecans are excellent nut choices. Just stay away from the salted and honey-roasted varieties.

Perk up dishes with the humble tomato

Tomato-based foods, like salsa, marinara sauce, and sun-dried tomatoes, can turn simple foods tantalizing, even when you give fat grams the heave-ho. Tangy salsa can replace high-fat gravies and sauces for meat and poultry.

It's also a succulent substitute for heavy baked potato toppings, like butter and sour cream. In addition, choose marinara dishes instead of alfredo or carbonara when eating Italian food. If you perk up dishes with the incredible taste of sun-dried tomatoes, you'll also get the cancer-fighting nutrient lycopene.

Food	Serving size	Fat grams saved by substituting marinara sauce
white sauce, medium, homemade	1/4 cup	6
cheese sauce, prepared from recipe	1/4 cup	8
mild nacho cheese sauce, ready-to-serve	1/4 cup	10
Food	**Serving size**	**Fat grams saved by substituting salsa**
sour cream, cultured	1 tbsp	3
butter, salted	1 tbsp	12

Fit in fish and chicken. Fish are particularly kind to your heart and may account for the unusually good health of people on the Mediterranean diet. Fatty fish, like salmon, trout, and herring, supply you with much-needed omega-3 fatty acids, a type of polyunsaturated fat. In addition, work in an occasional serving of skinless, low-fat poultry during the week.

Enjoy more olive oil. To the Greeks, this oil is almost a food group in itself. People from this part of the world often use it in place of other cooking oils, fats, butter, and dressings, and research suggests you should, too. Studies prove the monounsaturated fats in olive oil lower LDL and raise HDL cholesterol, clearing fat deposits out of your arteries and lowering your risk of heart attack.

It's not enough to simply add olive oil to your diet. You need to use it instead of harmful saturated and trans fats, like butter, margarine, shortening, lard, and corn oil. Extra virgin olive oil is the best kind. Make the switch, and you could be singing a happy 100th birthday to yourself.

Along with eating more whole grains, fruits and veggies, fish, and olive oil, you should reduce the amount of other items in your diet.

▶ Reduce the red meat. Plan beef and other red meats as a treat a few times a month. Skip fatty or processed meats, like sausage and bacon, and limit your eggs to just a few each week.

▶ Downplay dairy. If you lived in the Mediterranean region, you might eat more yogurt and cheese made from goat and sheep milk, which has a stronger flavor than that from cow's milk. Because of this fact, a little goes a long way. In fact, while Western diets emphasize dairy products for bone health, Greeks eat dairy more sparingly. This also cuts back on the saturated fat in their diet. You can keep your dairy by choosing low-fat versions, such as skim milk and nonfat yogurt. But learn to skip high-fat ice cream, cheese, and whole milk.

▶ Limit fats other than olive oil. Saturated and trans fats pose an alarming threat to your health. But they make up only a small amount of the energy, or calories, you eat each day on the Mediterranean diet. Cutting back on fatty meats; replacing butter and other fats with olive oil; and building meals out of whole, unprocessed plant foods goes a long way to putting a lid on saturated and trans fats in your diet.

▸ Say "no" to sweets. Sugary or fattening desserts and sweet snacks are the exception, not the rule, in a Mediterranean meal. You can enjoy them a few times a week as special treats, but try making fresh fruit your regular dessert.

▸ Limit your alcohol. No one needs to tell the Greeks to drink wine for their heart. They've been doing that for years. Moderate drinking – a glass of wine a day for women, and up to two a day for men – is a normal part of this diet. While heavy drinking is not a healthy habit, studies suggest moderate amounts of alcohol could reduce your risk of heart disease. If you're comfortable having a glass of wine with your meal, that's good news. But don't feel you must start drinking.

It may sound like all Greek people do is eat, but regular exercise is an integral part of their health. Take a cue from them and combine physical activity with your new Mediterranean eating plan. Your heart and your waistline will thank you.

Conquer a sweet tooth with pantry staple

Turn off your craving for sweets and help melt off pounds with this easy weight-loss secret. The next time your insatiable sweet tooth kicks in, just put this common household item on your tongue. Dissolve a teaspoon of baking soda in warm water, swish it around like mouthwash, then spit it out.

Small changes help you take off pounds

Sometimes it's the small things that trip you up on the path to your healthiest, most ideal weight. Avoid those pitfalls by using these helpful tips to change the way you live with food.

Make a smooth start. Stress can wreck your best intentions. If you are starting a new job, getting a divorce, or have experienced a recent death in your family, you might need to delay your plan to begin a diet. Give yourself more time to simply follow good eating habits without trying to lose weight. Then, when the stress has eased, you'll be ready to start cutting back on calories.

Choose a traditional dining spot. Make it a habit to sit down and eat at a table – not in the car, not at your desk at work, and not "on the run."

Dine amid soft or neutral colors. Bright colors stimulate the appetite, so choose calmer tones in tablecloths, napkins, and even dining room walls. Turning up the lights, on the other hand, may help you avoid overeating. One researcher found that people ate more in a darkened room.

Pick the perfect plate. Use a small dinner plate – the same size every meal. Helpings look larger on the smaller space, so you are less likely to overload or feel deprived. In addition, you'll need less measuring as you learn what a single serving of various foods looks like on your dish.

Take your time. Chew slowly and put down your fork between bites. Your brain needs 20 minutes to get the message your hunger is satisfied.

Play mellow music. Listening to soft classical music, according to one study, helps you eat less – and more slowly. But snappier rock 'n' roll may cause you to eat more and faster.

Stop eating when you're satisfied. When you reach that "had enough" feeling, put down your fork, get up from the table, put away leftovers, and get busy with something other than eating.

Stock up on healthy foods. Go through your pantry and refrigerator and remove all junk food. Restock your shelves with nutritious, low-calorie substitutes.

Calm down before you chow down. Don't turn to food to relieve tensions. If you are having a stressful day, go for a walk, meditate, or listen to soothing music to calm yourself before eating. You'll be less likely to overindulge.

Visualize success. Relax and use imagery each day to get a feel for victory. See yourself after you've reached your goal, slipping into a smaller-size outfit. Or imagine feeling proud as you step on your bathroom scale and see the lower number. Pretending it's already true enlists the support of your subconscious mind to make it really happen.

Take up a new – or rediscover an old – hobby. Choose a pastime, like knitting or cross-stitching. Hook a rug, put a puzzle together, or place family photos in an album. Not only will you keep your hands too busy to reach for a snack, but you'll also get the satisfaction of completing a task.

Measure your treats. Don't nibble from a bag or box, especially while watching television or using the computer. When you are distracted, you are likely to eat more than you planned. Instead, measure a small amount of food – like a handful of pretzels or a couple of cookies – and put the rest away. Give your full attention to slowly eating your snack before you return to your activity.

Drink up and freeze out fat. Some diet pros say drinking a big glass of ice water before meals will dull your appetite. Liquids of any temperature make you feel fuller. Besides that, sometimes people eat when they are really just thirsty. So pour a glass of water instead of reaching for something to nibble. If plain water seems boring, add a twist of lemon or drink flavored bottled water or unsweetened herbal iced tea.

Juice your way to a slim, trim figure. Delicious, vitamin-filled orange juice – or another fructose-rich juice – may be the perfect appetizer for anyone trying to lose weight. In a Yale study, those who drank a 200-calorie glass of juice half an hour or so before eating cut calories at mealtime – from 300 to more than 400 on average. Stir in a little pectin, used to thicken jams and jellies, and you may reduce your appetite even more.

Be positive about "negative" calories. Celery, cucumbers, and iceberg lettuce have very few calories. In fact, some people call them "negative-calorie" foods because, they say, in preparing, chewing, and digesting them, you burn more calories than they contain.

286

Whether or not this is true, snack away on them until you reach a healthy weight.

Eat light at night for a flat tummy. You may have heard that eating a big meal late at night isn't a good idea – whether you want to lose weight or just sleep well. But did you know this habit could give you a potbelly? That's because a heavy meal puts pressure on your stomach muscles and pushes them out. It does this more easily when these muscles are relaxed, as they are when you lie down to sleep. A "bay window" is the result if this happens regularly.

Worrying about your weight can also contribute to a bulging mid-section. Studies show stress seems to cause fat to settle around the waist – a dangerous place to carry it. Exercise, however, is helpful for both reducing stress and keeping pounds off. Try to hold your stomach muscles in when you walk, run, or do other exercises that bounce your belly. The flopping motion can weaken those abdominal muscles.

Shop with a list. Plan your meals carefully before you make your list for grocery shopping. Then stick to it while you are in the store. Don't linger in the aisles where you might be tempted to buy extras. Watch out, especially, for yummy-sounding names. Grandma's Oven-Fresh Old-Fashioned Oatmeal Cookies, for example, are probably plain oatmeal cookies, mass-produced in a commercial bakery. Remind yourself they are nothing special and go back to your list.

Read the labels. You'll learn a lot by reading the information on packages in the store. Better yet, many companies provide nutrition data – including calories – online. So surf for the facts before you make your shopping list.

Don't shop when you are hungry or rushed. Have a healthy, filling snack before you go out the door. The free food samples won't look so appetizing, and you'll be less tempted to buy unplanned extras from tantalizing displays. If you make it a leisurely shopping trip, you'll have time to compare brands for the lowest calories per serving. In addition, you'll have time to wait for the butcher to trim excess fat from the meats you buy.

Feast on foods that force weight loss. High-fiber fruits, vegetables, and grains are your most nutritious weight-loss foods. They eliminate snacking by filling your tummy with the fewest calories at mealtime. The fiber makes you feel so full, in fact, it's as if someone turned off your body's internal hunger switch. Moreover, most fiber actually passes through your system undigested, so you don't absorb all the calories. It does all this while lowering your cholesterol and blood pressure, too.

---

3 unusual causes of weight gain

Eating too much and not exercising are not always to blame for weight gain. If you stick to a moderate diet but the pounds still pile on, there could be another — although rare — explanation. Ask your doctor if one of these could be the cause.

Hypothyroidism. A thyroid that produces too little thyroid hormone may cause your metabolism to slow down so you gain weight. If this is your problem, you may often feel cold and fatigued. There's a blood test to check it out.

Genetics. You may have inherited a condition that contributes to weight gain, like not having enough of a particular hormone that signals when you are full.

Medications. Estrogen, some antidepressants, and several other drugs can cause weight gain. Don't stop taking your medication, but talk to your doctor about an alternative drug.

Check out the only 'diet' you'll ever need

After all the trendy diets you've tried, aren't you ready for an ultimate, sensible eating plan — one designed to help you maintain a healthy weight and prevent disease?

Several major health organizations — American Heart Association, American Cancer Society, American Dietetic Association, American

Academy of Pediatrics, and National Institutes of Health – joined forces to develop the Unified Dietary Guidelines.

These guidelines were designed to prevent disease by helping control obesity and encouraging you to eat a variety of healthy foods. Here are some of the recommendations:

▶ Fat. Eat no more than 20 to 35 percent of your total calories from all types of fat, including less than 10 percent from saturated fat.

▶ Cholesterol. You should limit dietary cholesterol to less than 300 milligrams (mg) a day. Keep trans fatty acid consumption as low as possible.

▶ Carbohydrates. Complex carbohydrates, such as cereals, grains, fruits, and vegetables, should make up 45 to 65 percent of your total daily calories.

▶ Salt. Your goal should be to eat less than 2,300 mg of sodium a day. That's approximately one teaspoon of salt.

▶ Calories. Don't consume more calories than you need to maintain a desirable body weight.

People with certain health conditions may have different needs, so you should check with your doctor before you change your diet. For example, the American Heart Association suggests that people with high cholesterol limit cholesterol in food to less than 200 mg a day.

Everyone needs a different number of calories to maintain weight or lose weight. A doctor could help you determine your specific needs – based on factors like your size, age, and activity level – but here are some examples:

If a 55-year-old woman who is 5'5" tall and weighs 135 pounds does four hours of very light activity, like reading or driving, and 30 minutes of light activity, like sweeping or walking, she would need 1,705 calories a day to maintain her current weight.

If a 55-year-old man who is 5'10" tall and weighs 155 pounds does four hours of very light activity and 30 minutes of light activity, he would need 1,975 calories to maintain his current weight.

The guidelines don't tell you exactly what to eat and how much, like most eating plans. Instead, you use your own judgment to stay within the guidelines. The best way to do this is to eat a variety of foods, especially foods from plant sources, like grains, fruits, and vegetables.

Delicious, low-fat dairy options

Try these tasty options to make low-fat dairy a part of your healthy diet.

▸ Switch to low-fat (1-percent) or nonfat (skim) milk instead of whole and reduced-fat (2-percent) milk.

▸ Look for low-fat cheeses with less than 3 grams of fat per ounce. Cut down on full-fat, processed, and hard cheeses, like American, cheddar, and brie.

▸ Use soft margarines. The softer they are, the less saturated fat they contain. Try tubs and tubes of margarine or vegetable oil spread.

▸ Buy margarine that lists a vegetable oil as its first ingredient. Steer clear of those made with hydrogenated or partially hydrogenated oils.

▸ Forget sour cream — use plain, low-fat yogurt instead.

Get milk and get slim

Can you drink milk and lose weight? Some research shows adding calcium to your diet can help you lose weight — if you do it wisely. Drinking this all-natural, nutrient-loaded beverage three times a day may help you shed some fat.

Dr. Robert Heaney, with the Osteoporosis Research Center of Creighton University, found that women with low calcium levels were more than twice as likely to be overweight. Then, in a group of 780 dieters, those who got the most calcium lost more weight than those without extra calcium. Perhaps more importantly, other research indicates a calcium-rich diet means you'll lose body fat, not lean muscle.

Animal research at the University of Tennessee, conducted by Dr. Michael Zemel, discovered that a low-calorie, high-dairy diet caused a loss of up to 70 percent of body fat. Low-calorie, low-calcium diets only reduced fat by 8 percent.

Both Zemel and Heaney think that calcium helps control how you burn fat. When your calcium levels are low, your body thinks you're starving, so it stores fat. When they are high, it burns fat more efficiently. In other words, you may be able to raise your metabolism and drop pounds with calcium.

Zemel has done other studies on dairy and weight, including one of overweight people who cut 500 calories from their daily diet and added calcium in various forms. One group took daily calcium supplements, while another group added three servings of dairy products to their diet. A third group took a placebo. After about six months, the people on the dairy diet had lost the most weight — nearly 11 percent of their body weight.

But not everyone agrees that milk is the ticket to weight-loss success. Many clinical human studies have been too small, too short, or funded by the dairy industry. That's why large clinical trials and further research are still needed to help settle issues like how calcium affects weight, how safe and effective it may be, and the best way to use it. Because the jury is still out on the calcium–weight loss connection, the Federal Trade Commission recently ruled dairy producers must stop claiming their products cause weight loss until research provides stronger evidence.

Bump up your numbers. More than half of all adults in the United States don't get the recommended amount of calcium — which the National Academy of Sciences has set at 1,000 to 1,200 milligrams (mg) a day for seniors. Adding just one to two servings of dairy (from 300 to 600 mg of calcium) to your diet every day may make a difference in your weight.

Watch the fat. Remember that calcium is no magic diet pill. It only helps you lose weight if you're already on a reduced-calorie diet. So add calcium-rich dairy to your meals only if you cut calories somewhere else.

According to the Virginia Cooperative Extension Service, calcium choices can vary greatly in their fat content. Go for the lower fat options.

Dig into dairy. Here are some easy ways to include dairy foods in a low-calorie diet.

▶ Add low-fat milk to your coffee and tea.

▶ Cook warm cereals with low-fat milk instead of water.

▶ Substitute a smoothie blended with fruit, ice, and low-fat milk for that high-calorie milk shake.

▶ Treat yourself to half a cup of low-fat frozen yogurt.

▶ Add two servings of low-fat yogurt to your daily menu. Mix in some fruit for a yummy dessert.

▶ Bake with milk instead of water, except yeast breads.

▶ Sprinkle fat-free dry milk powder on almost anything. You won't notice the taste or calories, and 2 tablespoons add about 100 extra milligrams of calcium.

Hunt down other sources. If you're lactose intolerant or don't like milk, you can still beef up on calcium without dairy.

▶ While calcium supplements are only about half as effective as dairy in helping you lose weight, you can try a daily dose of around 500 mg of calcium citrate.

▶ Canned sardines and salmon with bones are calcium-rich. So are broccoli, rutabagas, and Chinese cabbage. Dark-green, leafy vegetables, like collards, turnip greens, kale, and spinach, are also rich in calcium, but they contain oxalic acid, which interferes with your body's ability to absorb calcium.

▶ Some packaged foods also have added calcium. Fortified orange juice can have almost as much calcium as milk.

Enriched cereals, soy-based foods, canned tomatoes, and stone-ground flour can all have calcium added during processing. Read nutrition labels for your best sources.

Keep in mind that calcium is only a small piece of the big diet puzzle. It can help your body lose weight, but not on its own.

Go high in calcium, low in fat						
Calcium (mg)	Low-fat food choice	Fat (g)	Medium-fat food choice	Fat (g)	High-fat food choice	Fat (g)
300	1 cup skim milk	0	1 cup whole milk	8	1 cup eggnog	19
200	1 oz low-fat cheese	6	1 oz American cheese	9	1/8 of 8″ Quiche Lorraine	39
100	4″ pancake	4	7″ waffle	11	1 cup commercial granola	20

Take a look at the latest food label lingo

Nutrition information on food labels appears in a standard form, but it may still be confusing. To help you out, the government has established definitions for terms used on food labels. Learn these terms so you know what you're getting.

Serving size. The size may be much smaller or much larger than what you consider a single serving. Remember this when reading any figures that explain calories or nutrients per serving.

Fat-free. Contains less than 0.5 grams (g) of fat per serving.

Sugar-free. Has less than 0.5 g of sugar per serving. But the term "low sugar" is not regulated and may or may not mean what you expect.

Low-fat. Contains no more than 3 g of fat per serving.

Good source of calcium. Must have at least 100 milligrams (mg) of calcium per serving. A good source of a nutrient must have 10 to 19 percent of the recommended daily value. An excellent source must have at least 20 percent.

Light or lite. Has one-third fewer calories or half the fat of the higher-calorie, higher-fat food. This could also mean the item has half the sodium of a low-calorie, low-fat food.

Lean. Contains less than 10 g of fat, 4 g of saturated fat, and 95 mg of cholesterol per serving of fish, poultry, or meat.

Reduced. Has at least 25 percent less fat, saturated fat, sodium, cholesterol, sugar, or calories per serving than the regular food.

Watch your beverage to watch your waistline

Drink	Calories	Minutes of brisk walking to burn those calories *
skim milk (8 oz.)	83	12 minutes
hot cocoa (6 oz.)	113	17 minutes
whole milk (8 oz.)	146	22 minutes
unsweetened grape juice (8 oz.)	154	23 minutes
cola (12 oz.)	155	23 minutes
vanilla milkshake (11 oz.)	351	53 minutes
chocolate milkshake (11 oz.)	357	54 minutes

* Times are approximate. The number of calories burned depends on several factors, including weight, workout intensity, and fitness level.

Secret weapon in the war on fat

Watching what you eat will help you take off extra weight. But that's only part of the story. The other part is getting physically active – that's right – exercise.

Physical activity is a double-barreled weapon in the fight to be fit. It helps you burn more calories, and it also builds muscle, which burns calories faster than fat tissue. On top of that, people who exercise are more likely to stick to a weight-loss plan.

Getting active doesn't have to be painful. In fact, a brisk walk might help you shed more pounds than a fast run, according to research in Greece. In the three-month study, 14 women who exercised at a moderate pace lost more weight than the women who exercised more vigorously. The researchers suggest striving for a combination of moderate and vigorous exercise – with your doctor's approval – for the most benefits. When you exercise strenuously, you rev up your metabolism, and you'll continue to burn more calories long after you stop exercising.

Try a treadmill. If you are thinking about buying an exercise machine, consider this – the best choice for burning calories is a treadmill. Wear your walking shoes when you shop for a treadmill so you can try it out in the store. Make sure the controls and handrails are located comfortably and the belt fits your stride. You can probably get along fine with a less-durable, and less-expensive, treadmill if you are using it for walking only rather than running. Hop on for 10 minutes at a time about four times a day for the best results.

Lift some weight. Resistance, or strength, training is a great way to replace fat with muscle. You can do these exercises at home with equipment ranging from simple household items to sophisticated gear from a sporting goods store. You can also join a health club or fitness center for access to a wider range of equipment and trainers to help you decide the exact exercises you need.

Act your age. People age 55 and older account for about 25 percent of all gym and health club memberships, and many programs are designed for middle-age and older adults. One program, available to people who have reached 65 years, is the SilverSneakers Fitness Program. Benefits include a free membership at a participating fitness center and exercise classes geared for seniors. Leading Medicare health plans and Medicare Supplement carriers offer the program at no extra cost. For more information, call 888-423-4632 toll free or visit *www.silversneakers.com* on the Internet.

Amazing nut makes a great low-fat snack

A single chocolate chip cookie contains 13 times as much fat as one chestnut, and it has twice as many calories. So if you need a lightweight snack that won't leave you starving for junk food, chestnuts are worth a try.

Don't worry about the high fat content of nuts. This one is different. As the following table shows, most nuts weigh in with five to 10 times as many fat grams as chestnuts. Fresh chestnuts are available from September through February. Pick the ones that feel firm to the touch.

Nut	Number of nuts per 1-ounce serving	Fat grams per 1-ounce serving
chestnuts	12 to 13	2
pistachios	49	13
cashews	18	13
almonds	24	14
peanuts	28	14
hazelnuts	20	17
walnuts	7	18
pecans	10	20
macadamia nuts	10 to 12	22

Get the skinny on popular diet plans

It's easy to find a diet plan that will knock off several pounds fairly quickly, but the trick is keeping off those pounds for good. In a recent study, researchers concluded it doesn't make much difference which diet plan you use as long as you stick with it.

The study results showed weight loss was about the same for the Atkins, Ornish, Weight Watchers, and the Zone diet plans. Unfortunately, only 50 to 65 percent of the participants stayed with their diets for the full year of the study. Here's a look at some of the most popular diet plans.

▶ Restricted calories. The more you cut calories, the faster you'll lose weight. But watch out for cutting back too much. Extreme diets of fewer than 1,100 calories can have serious health consequences, and you're more likely to binge or overeat when you go off the diet.

▶ High protein, low carbohydrate. These diets are proving to be effective for short-term weight loss, but experts are concerned about their long-term effects on your health. The Atkins diet emphasizes high-protein and low-carbohydrate intake, while the South Beach and the Zone diets allow certain types of carbs.

▶ Low-fat, high fiber. This approach is to replace fat with complex carbohydrates, like fruits, vegetables, and whole grains. You count grams of fat instead of calories. But when you eliminate fat, you may miss out on some important nutrients. Commercial "low-fat" products are also likely to be loaded with sugar and other ingredients with no nutritional value.

The simplest and least expensive weight-loss plan is to cut back on calories and exercise for at least 30 minutes a day, five times a week. Cutting fat, protein, or carbohydrates may make a diet fashionable or easy to follow, but it only works when you burn more calories than you take in. Depending on your age, sex, and activity level, you need 12 to 15 calories a day per pound of your desired weight.

To lose weight – and keep it off – find a plan you'll stick with. It should give you proper nutrition yet allow you to control your calories. You could also work to make healthy food choices rather than following a strict diet. No matter what plan you choose, make sure you find time to exercise.

Simple secret of successful dieters

"Eat breakfast yourself, share lunch with a friend, and give dinner away to your enemy." This old Russian proverb would be a great motto for people battling the bulge. Eating breakfast helps you lose weight – and keep it off. Nearly four out of five people in the National Weight Control Registry, a survey of almost 3,000 people who have lost at least 30 pounds and kept it off for a year or more, eat breakfast every day.

The right kind of breakfast keeps you from getting hungry and loading up on calories later in the day. Choose whole grain cereals and fruit, but steer clear of sugary cereals. Sugar, a simple carbohydrate, raises your blood sugar quickly – then it falls, and you're hungry again. Both whole grains and eggs, another breakfast favorite, will help you feel full longer.

Back to basics — simple slimming solutions

Weight-loss tips are as numerous as the tempting choices on a church dinner's dessert table. It's hard to sort through all that advice to separate gimmicks from truly great ideas. Here are some basic changes you can make to control your weight.

Break your fast. A good time to eat the majority of your calories is in the morning. Adults who eat breakfast every day tend to weigh less and have lower cholesterol levels. Also, the body's ability to burn calories is greater in the morning than in the afternoon or evening. People who skip breakfast tend to eat more high-fat snacks, too. Some nutrition specialists recommend that 20 to 25 percent of your daily calories come from breakfast. This is also a good meal to focus on fruit.

Turn off the tube. Don't eat while watching television. The average person eats eight times more food watching prime-time TV than at any other time.

Consider chromium. Chromium appears to aid weight loss by burning fat more quickly as well as helping your body build muscle. Chromium also works with insulin in the body to keep blood sugar levels even, so your energy level remains stable and you burn food more efficiently.

Get your chromium from food rather than from dietary supplements, because the jury is still out on the possible benefits of supplemental chromium. Some good sources include apples with skins, asparagus, liver, mushrooms, nuts, prunes, oysters, fish, and other seafood.

Make healthy choices if you're a nighttime eater. It's not when you eat that counts as much as what you eat. No doubt you've heard everything you eat after 8 p.m. goes straight to your hips. Well, a new study says it's just not so. Researchers found a calorie counts the same no matter when you eat it. However, women who ate most of their calories at night got less vitamin C, vitamin B6, folic acid, and carbohydrates from their diet than women who spread their calories out over the day. Nighttime eaters also were more likely to get more calories from fat, protein, and alcohol. This could be because they were so hungry by the time they ate they made poor nutritional choices.

Count both calories and fat grams. Even though it would be easier to count only one or the other, research suggests you'll get better results from your weight-loss efforts if you count both.

A study from Indiana University found that overweight people ate about the same number of calories as lean people. However, the plump people ate more fat and added sugar while the lean people ate more fiber. This seems to suggest that you can eat more food if you change the form of the calories from fat and sugar to fiber.

Although Americans have significantly reduced their fat intake in recent years, they're still packing on extra pounds. Thinking that low-fat or fat-free means low-calorie, Americans are eating too many calories. If you eat more calories than you need — whether from fat or from carbohydrates — your body stores them as fat.

Don't skip meals. Meal-skipping is a big factor in falling off the diet bandwagon and into an eating binge. Giving your body fuel at regular intervals keeps blood sugar levels stable and helps your body burn calories more efficiently.

Watch yourself in social situations. People eat more when they are with other people, says a study at Georgia State University. When you're counting calories, be careful when eating in a group.

Tailor your diet. Everyone is different, so your weight-loss regimen should match your own style of eating. If you are a constant nibbler, plan healthy meals and snacks ahead of time to meet your calorie goals. If you eat more when you're bored or frustrated, plan pleasant activities to distract you from overeating. If the vending machines at work are a constant temptation, take healthy snacks with you from home.

Make your cheddar better. Don't want to give up your favorite high-fat cheese? Make a low-fat version by zapping it in the microwave for a minute or two. Heating will make the fat separate somewhat from the cheese. Any oil you can pour or blot off will significantly reduce the cheese's fat content. This method also works well for pizzas, fajitas, cheese sandwiches, or cheese toppings on casseroles.

The inside story on dietary fats

Your body needs some fats to stay healthy. They provide the raw materials for making hormones and bile. Other fats carry the fat-soluble vitamins — A, D, E, and K — in your bloodstream throughout your body.

12 smart ways to eat less fat

Part of a successful weight-loss plan is learning how to live a low-fat lifestyle. Not only are low-fat foods healthier for your body, but going low-fat lets you eat a little more food without a lot more calories. That's because fats contain nine calories per gram, while all carbohydrates and proteins contain four calories per gram. That means fat has more than double the calories of the other major nutrients.

The best news of all is that low-fat living doesn't have to be a tedious, torturous ordeal. In fact, studies show as you reduce the amount of fat you eat, your cravings for fatty foods actually decline. Researchers at the Fred Hutchinson Cancer Research Center in Seattle found that people who switch from high-fat to low-fat foods soon develop a preference for lower-fat foods.

Here are some tips to help you make a smooth transition to a low-fat lifestyle.

▶ Use low-fat or nonfat dairy foods to replace cream in sauces. Substitute skim milk for whole milk.

▶ Steam, poach, roast, broil, grill, microwave, or bake foods rather than sauté or pan-fry them. Cook meat on a rack so the fat drains off.

▶ Skim the fat off soups or stews. If possible, cook the broth in advance, chill it, then remove the hardened layer of fat on top.

▶ Season vegetables with herbs, spices, chicken broth, or lemon juice instead of high-fat butter and sauces. Experiment with new seasonings.

▶ Perk up flavors with balsamic vinegar, sun-dried tomatoes, Dijon mustard, Tabasco sauce, salsa, catsup, green chilies, or small amounts of sesame or hot chili oils.

▶ Make your own reduced-fat dressing by using more vinegar and less oil. Use lemon juice and Italian herbs for fat-free flavor. When buying mayonnaise, opt for the reduced-fat or fat-free version.

▸ Cut back the fat in your favorite recipes by one-third and replace the fat in baked recipes with applesauce or puréed prunes.

▸ Take advantage of healthful cookware, such as microwave ovens, vegetable steamers, pressure cookers, and nonstick pots and pans. Using these tools to cook helps preserve nutrients and makes cooking a little easier as well.

▸ Limit eating red meat and other animal products to once or twice a week. When choosing meat, keep in mind that those cuts labeled "select" tend to be lowest in fat. Always trim away fatty edges and remove skin from chicken before cooking.

▸ Substitute olive or canola oil for other vegetable fats.

▸ Go for burgers made without grease. Microwave your patties for one to three minutes; pour off the liquid; and then fry, broil, or grill them. This cuts the fat content by almost one-third.

▸ Buy tuna packed in water instead of oil.

Wash away pounds with water

Fill yourself up with a tall, shimmering glass of water, and you'll be less likely to overeat, say some experts. Research suggests that drinking about six cups of water a day could raise your metabolic rate — the rate at which you burn calories. But don't overdo it. Drinking too much water can be harmful.

In one study, drinking cold water after a meal led to an increase in fat burning in men, while in women, drinking water increased carbohydrate burning.

Nobody is really sure whether or not simply drinking water will make you shed pounds, but if you choose water instead of high-calorie drinks, you may be amazed at the results. For a delicious change of pace, experiment with a splash of fruit juice in your water or a tangy squeeze from a lemon or lime.

Think small for big changes

Little changes in lifestyle can add up to big changes in weight. That should be encouraging news to anyone struggling with weight loss. Every time you pass up dessert – every time you park a little farther from the store – you're adding fuel to your personal weight-loss fire. Here are a few more examples of small but helpful changes anyone can make.

Fidget. Your mom probably taught you not to fidget. But new studies suggest that people who fidget burn more calories than people who don't. Researchers call this "fidget factor" NEAT (nonexercise activity thermogenesis) and say it accounts for an average of 348 calories burned in a day.

Tapping your toes or drumming your fingers may be annoying to the people around you, but if you do it when you're alone, you could burn off some extra pounds with very little effort.

Eat in. If you limit how often you eat out, you may save money and lose weight. A recent study found the more often people ate in restaurants, the more overweight they were likely to be. Researchers theorize that the increase in restaurant eating in the United States could be responsible in part for the national rise in the number of obese people.

Keep it small. According to a recent survey by the American Institute for Cancer Research, people in the United States believe that, when it comes to weight control, the kind of food they eat is more important than how much. The survey also found people underestimate portion size. Although the kind of food you eat is important, eating too much of any food – even low-fat foods – adds unnecessary calories and weight.

One way to keep your portions under control is to buy smaller containers of food. A University of Chicago at Urbana-Champaign researcher found that when people ate popcorn from a large container, they consumed 44 percent more than people who were eating from smaller containers. If you buy food in small containers rather than the jumbo economy size, you may eat less. While you're working on smaller portions, you might also try using smaller plates. A small plate will look full with less food.

Each of these small changes may not make a huge and immediate difference in your weight. But if you make several small changes and give it time, you may be pleasantly surprised by the difference you'll see.

Trick your body into losing weight

People tend to eat the same amount of food, regardless of calories. So instead of trying to limit how much you eat, pay attention to your food's energy density. That means the number of calories in each gram. The more fiber or water in a food, the lower its energy (or calorie) density. You'll feel more satisfied while eating fewer calories.

For example, soups have a low energy density because of their high water content. Vegetables are less energy dense than, say pasta. Another trick is to beat foods. Turn ice cream into a milkshake to add air, and you'll be more satisfied with less. By choosing low-energy-dense foods, you could lose weight while eating as much — or more — than you do now.

Dine out without throwing out your diet

Americans are getting bigger, and they're big into eating out. That's probably no coincidence. A recent study found the more often people ate in restaurants, the more overweight they were likely to be. Researchers theorize that the increase in restaurant eating in the United States could be responsible in part for the national rise in obesity statistics.

But you don't need to completely avoid restaurants because you're trying to lose weight. Go with a plan, or the menu will sabotage your best intentions. These tips should help you enjoy the experience — and stick to your calorie count.

Opt for lunch. The portions are generally smaller than at dinner.

Go light. Choose a restaurant with "light" dishes on the menu. Or call ahead to see if they will make adjustments, like grilling an item that's usually fried or substituting steamed vegetables for french fries.

Divide and conquer. Ask for a take-out container at the beginning rather than the end of a meal. Fill it with half your food – two-thirds if the restaurant serves extra-large portions – before you begin to eat. You can divide the food again when you get home, then freeze or refrigerate it for later meals.

Skip the entrees. Instead, make your meal from a salad, broth-based soup, and a low-calorie appetizer – like shrimp cocktail.

Ban the buffet. If you can't avoid an all-you-can-eat food bar, limit yourself to two trips. Load up a dinner plate with fruits, salads, and other low-calorie vegetable dishes. If you eat it all and still want more, use a small salad plate for the second visit.

Allow sensible treats. When a pizza craving hits, order a veggie special on thin crust with double tomato sauce and a light sprinkling of cheese.

Know your fares. Ethnic restaurants can have baffling menus. To figure out which dishes won't add to your weight, look for these menu tip-offs.

▸ Italian. Stay away from Alfredo, carbonara, parmigiana, and anything that's stuffed or fried. Choose entrees described as primavera, piccata, marinara, grilled, or thin crust.

▸ Chinese. Crispy, crunchy, sweet and sour, and fried dishes are all loaded with calories. Look for steamed dishes and ones containing these words – jum, kow, and shu.

▸ Mexican. Eat nachos, chimichangas, guacamole, and taco salad shells only rarely. But you can fill up on fajitas, entrees with shredded meat, soft corn tortillas, salsa, rice, or black beans.

▶ French. Lovely as they are, limit entrees with these words – pâté, crème, au gratin, fromage, hollandaise, en croute, béarnaise, mousse, foie gras, or pastry. Instead, enjoy the delicate flavor of fruit sauces and choose poached, roasted, or en papillote dishes.

▶ Indian, Thai, and Island fare. Limit the amount of fritters and coconut dishes, and indulge in marinated, steamed, stir-fried, tandoori, Tikka, and satay dishes.

Fast-food champs and chumps

It's best to eat at home when you're trying to control your weight. If you must eat out, fast food is usually not the best option. But sometimes it's the only meal in a pinch. Learn how to make good choices when you go out.

Restaurant	Steer clear	Better bet
Arby's	Bac'n Cheddar Deluxe (539 calories)	Grilled Chicken BBQ (388 calories)
McDonald's	Big Mac (560 calories)	Grilled chicken salad deluxe, fat-free herb vinaigrette dressing (170 calories)
Pizza Hut	Pepperoni Personal Pan Pizza (670 calories)	Thin 'N Crispy Veggie Lover's Pizza, two slices (340 calories)
Taco Bell	Nachos BellGrande (770 calories)	Grilled chicken soft taco (240 calories)
Wendy's	Chicken club sandwich (470 calories)	Grilled chicken Caesar salad, fat-free French dressing (295 calories)

Fool yourself into shedding pounds

The best eating plan is one you don't have to think about. Too many food choices and dieting decisions mean more chances to slip up. So make it easy on yourself, and set up your surroundings to help you lose weight without effort.

One way to fool yourself is make small portions of food look bigger. Years of study show it's not how much you eat that makes you feel full but how much you think you have eaten. By fooling your eyes into seeing portions as larger than they actually are, you can trick your stomach into feeling full with less food. Experts say trimming just 15 to 20 percent of your daily calories this way could help you lose 30 pounds in a year, without hardly trying.

Downsize your dishes. Use smaller plates and bowls at home. Bigger dishes create an optical illusion, so a normal-size scoop of food that fills a small plate looks lost on a big one. If a portion looks too small to your eyes, your stomach assumes it is, prompting you to eat more.

Even food experts fall for this trick. In one sneaky study, nutrition experts ate 30 percent more ice cream when they scooped it into extra-large bowls than they did using regular-size bowls. Similarly, when you serve yourself from a huge bowl or platter, you tend to take and eat more food than usual. Try substituting salad plates for your regular plates and serving meals from smaller platters and bowls.

Shrink your spoons. The size of your utensils matters, too. The ice cream–eating researchers dished up almost 15 percent more when they used large scoops compared to small ones. In another study, people were allowed to serve themselves as many M&M candies as they wanted. Halfway through the study, researchers swapped the small serving spoon in the bowl with a large one. People who used the big spoon ate twice as much candy. So while trading in your big dishes, hunt for smaller silverware, too, and make a point of serving meals with smaller spoons, scoops, and forks.

Go skinny with glasses. Drink high-calorie beverages like soda and alcohol from tall, slim glasses rather than short, wide ones, and you will automatically drink about 30 percent less. Short, wide glasses look like they hold less, so you tend to pour more into them than you think.

Plump up your food. The way you prepare the food you eat can trick your stomach just as surely as the size plates you use. People who normally ate a half-pound hamburger were given a quarter-pound burger dressed up with lots of lettuce, onion, and tomatoes to make it look as big as the half-pound burger. These hungry people felt just as full after eating the smaller burger as they did after eating the big one, but they consumed fewer calories. Whipping foods to make them fuller and thicker has the same stomach-fooling effect.

Make things easy on yourself

As with everything, there is a good way and a bad way to shape up. You can try to change your lifetime habits through willpower, but that's difficult. Temptation is everywhere, and it can be very difficult to change your routine. In fact, one study of theatergoers found they were so used to eating during a movie, they even chowed down on stale, five-day-old popcorn. The popcorn was so old, researchers decided they must have been snacking out of habit.

Develop a plan with specific strategies to change your habits in small ways. For example, instead of dining out at an all-you-can-eat buffet, try a restaurant that offers smaller portions or tasty low-fat options. If you love cherry cheesecake, buy one slice but don't bring the whole cheesecake home. You won't fall into the habit of polishing off those high-calorie leftovers later.

5 clever ways to eat less

Weight-loss pills may sound like the answer to your prayers, but these drugs can do more harm than good, not to mention costing you an arm and a leg. And single-food diets promising miracles can be nutritional nightmares. What you need are some healthy tricks that will melt off those pounds naturally and easily.

Lean on low-density foods. Here's a trick that will allow you to eat the same amount of food, feel just as full, but absorb fewer calories. The scientific fact behind this "magic" is food density — the amount of calories a food has per portion. Low-density foods, like fruits and vegetables, are bulky and filling, but they don't carry a lot of calories. High-density foods, on the other hand, have a ton of calories crammed into small servings, mainly because they are loaded with fats and sugars.

To see the difference, try substituting the same amount of a low-density food for a high-density food — say 3 ounces of strawberries for 3 ounces of potato chips. You'll find you feel just as satisfied with the fruit, probably even more so. On top of that, you'll save yourself hundreds of calories.

Your goal is to eat more low-density foods, such as produce, whole grains, and legumes, and cut down on fatty, sugary foods. But remember — even low-fat or fat-free snacks can be high-density because of their tremendous sugar content.

Fluff up your food. You may remember adding Fluff to your peanut butter sandwiches as a child. That sugary confection will not help you lose weight, but food with extra air whipped in just might. A study at Pennsylvania State University found these "fluffy" foods could help you eat less.

In the study, 28 men drank one of three different kinds of milkshakes before lunch. All three milkshakes had the same ingredients, but some were blended longer to add air and volume. The men who drank the "airy" shakes ate 12 percent fewer calories at lunch, and they did not make up for it by eating more at dinner. If you must snack, trick your senses by filling up on an air-filled treat, like low-fat frozen yogurt or butter-free popcorn.

Shrink your serving sizes. Cleaning your plate could be one of the only bad habits your mom taught you. This is especially true if you eat at a typical restaurant with a mountain of food on your platter. According to a recent study, the more you have on your plate, the more you'll eat. Fortunately, the opposite is true as well.

One great way to limit your serving size is to cook at home, where you can control how much food you cook. You also can try eating off a smaller plate to reduce the size of your portions. Things get trickier when you eat out, but there are ways around a restaurant's generosity. Overcome huge entrees by splitting them with your spouse or friend. If you go it alone, put half your dinner into a doggie bag before you even start eating. That way, you won't be tempted by a full plate.

Limit food variety. A wide selection of food may be appealing when you're at a buffet, but it won't be when you get on the scale afterward. An overload of food appears to make your stomach's fuel gauge shut down. You're more likely to go beyond "full" just so you can taste everything. Experts think this tendency comes from our ancestors, who had to eat a variety of foods to guarantee they got all their nutrients.

The trick is to limit your snack selection. Store only one brand of chips in your cupboard or one type of cake in your fridge. You'll end up snacking less often because you'll get tired of the same old taste. On the other hand, stockpile a wide selection of fruits and vegetables. Variety in this case means getting a mix of nutrients and natural phytochemicals that would make your ancestors envious.

Ditch high-calorie drinks. You've heard of a beer belly, but how about a soda belly? Experts say you can put on pounds without realizing it by drinking high-calorie beverages. Your body doesn't seem to register the drinks because they go right through you. So you take in hundreds of empty calories, and your stomach is still hungry for more.

Do yourself a favor, and replace most of your high-calorie drinks with low- or no-calorie ones, like tea and water. You'll quench your thirst and save some pounds.

Cast off extra pounds with salmon

Heard that old joke about the seafood diet? "Every time I see food, I eat it." There's a real seafood diet that may work. Not only is salmon delicious, but it also contains a special fat that might help you lose weight. One study found eating a daily serving of fish high in omega-3 fatty acids helped people lose an extra 4 pounds during a 16-week study. The fact that omega-3 fatty acids in your diet may also keep your heart healthy, ward off some forms of cancer, protect your vision, and keep your brain sharp makes fish a great catch.

Just be picky about the fish you eat. Whether shopping for fish or eating out, choose wisely to limit your mercury and polychlorinated biphenyls (PCBs) exposure. Avoid tilefish, shark, swordfish, and king mackerel. Good choices include salmon, herring, sardines, shad, trout, mackerel, and whitefish.

According to the U.S. Department of Agriculture, farm-raised salmon have fewer omega-3 fatty acids than wild salmon. Experts have also found higher levels of dangerous contaminants, like PCBs, in farm-raised fish. The contaminants come from the food the fish eat in captivity. If you want the most benefits, stick with the wild varieties. These are often inexpensive. Virtually all canned salmon and mackerel are wild.

Dig up the 'dirt' on weight-loss gimmicks

Losing weight is tough, so it's good to know what might be holding you back. If you are trying to shrink your waistline, but you're plagued by weight-loss attempts that fail, consider the following information.

▶ Low-fat food labeling can cause problems. Labels can be deceiving, so make sure you check the calorie content. Another problem with low-fat foods is they tend to be less filling, so people eat more — and even then they are not satisfied.

▶ Drinking a smoothie with your meal is no bargain. Smoothies can be high in calories. It might be best to think of a smoothie as a healthy meal itself rather than a drink to go with your meal or snack.

▶ Eating out can mean pigging out. Portions in restaurants can be out of control. Eat at restaurants that serve smaller portions or put half your order in a to-go container before you start eating.

▶ Don't settle in for a meal or snack in front of the tube. Research has found that television distracts you from feeling full, which can lead to overeating.

▶ Low-carb or carb-free liquor labeling can be misleading. Beer and wine contain sugar and that means calories. Watch your calories when it comes to the liquor you drink.

▶ Alcohol consumption can affect weight and liver health. The liver secretes bile and bile breaks down fat molecules. That's why alcohol consumption can add up to abdominal weight gain.

Pick your 'label' for a slimmer identity

Do you have a taste for good food and drink? Can you spot the differences among fine cheeses, chocolates, or coffees? Then you may be a gourmet — a person with discriminating taste in food and wine. If you're watching your weight, that's a better label for yourself than gourmand. This food-lover also appreciates good food. The difference is, a gourmand loves to indulge in great quantities. You could even call him a glutton. So go ahead — be a gourmet and love your food. Just do it within reason.

Weigh the benefits of green tea

Green tea is known for fighting cancer and heart and respiratory disease, and many people claim its fat-fighting properties make it a natural complement to any healthy weight-loss program.

Some studies suggest the antioxidants in green tea, called catechin polyphenols, might help with weight loss by restricting the activity of amylase, a carbohydrate-digesting enzyme in saliva. Researchers think this action may slow the digestion of carbohydrates, which prevents the sudden rise of insulin in the blood and makes you burn fat instead of storing it. Others suggest the polyphenols in green tea increase your metabolism to help you burn extra calories.

Extract beats brew. In 1985, French researchers conducted one of the first trials on green tea's effect on fat. The study involved 60 middle-age obese women who started a diet of 1,800 calories a day and took green tea extract at each meal for 30 days.

After two weeks, the green tea group lost twice as much weight as those on the same diet who took a placebo instead. After four weeks, the green tea group had lost three times as much weight as the placebo group. This group also enjoyed significantly greater losses in waist size.

More studies have been done since 1985, but most have focused on how many calories green tea extract burns, which doesn't always mean the same thing as losing weight.

The National Institutes of Health sponsored one of the most recent studies. In this study, 70 moderately obese adults took two capsules of green tea extract twice a day, containing a daily total of 375 milligrams of catechin. After three months, their body weight dropped 4.6 percent (that's almost 10 pounds if you began at 200) and 4.48 percent off their waist (2.25 inches if you began at 50 inches).

But here's the catch. You can melt pounds away with green tea, but not by drinking it. You would have to drink an awful lot of green tea to get the dose of fat-burning ingredients the participants in these trials received. They weren't drinking green tea. They were getting large doses of its active ingredients in green tea extract capsules.

Drink to good health. There's no question about it. Green tea's health benefits are amazing. But its usefulness as an aid to weight loss is clearly complementary — it helps. It complements a nutritious diet with limited portions and a daily exercise plan. So don't put your hopes for a dramatic drop in weight in green tea alone.

One more caution — unless the green tea you use is clearly marked "decaffeinated," it will contain caffeine. Although green tea has less caffeine than black tea and about one-third as much as coffee, too much might keep you awake at night or make you feel nervous. If this is true for you, switch to decaffeinated green tea. You can also buy decaffeinated green tea extract.

Add some spice to your life

You can turn low-cal dishes into high-flavor international cuisine with versatile spices. Plain beans turn interesting when you add taste-boosters like rosemary, summer savory, or marjoram. The American Heart Association also recommends these delightful seasonings for veggies — chives, cider vinegar, garlic, onion, paprika, or parsley.

Powerful protectors
When diet and exercise aren't enough

Zap cholesterol with psyllium

Here's good news if controlling cholesterol is a major concern for you. Psyllium, the active ingredient in bulk laxatives, like Metamucil, Fiberall, Modane Bulk Powder, or Serutan, can help regulate cholesterol and battle blood sugar. In fact, one study suggests this natural substance lowers LDL cholesterol levels by up to 13 percent – and blood sugar levels by almost 20 percent.

Evicts cholesterol three ways. Psyllium is a super source of soluble fiber. So it can sop up cholesterol-containing bile salts and sweep them through your intestines and out of your body. As a result, your body must produce new bile acids from its cholesterol stores in the liver. Pulling from these reserves lowers cholesterol.

Psyllium probably also cuts your cholesterol in two other ways – by reducing the amount of fat and cholesterol you absorb from food and by inhibiting your liver's ability to produce cholesterol.

Dozens of clinical trials have shown psyllium lowers total and LDL cholesterol. In fact, the FDA has approved the following health claim, "Diets low in saturated fat and cholesterol that include soluble fiber from psyllium seed husk may reduce the risk of heart disease."

Siphons off blood sugar. Once in your digestive system, psyllium forms a gel that slows the digestion of food as it moves through your system. Because it takes longer to break down carbohydrates and absorb blood sugar into your bloodstream, insulin has more time to convert that blood sugar into energy.

In fact, a small study of 20 men and women with diabetes reported encouraging results. After taking 14 grams of psyllium daily for six weeks, study participants cut their average blood sugar absorption by 12 percent. However, results varied greatly between individuals. Their total and LDL cholesterol also dropped significantly. Then again, not all studies are positive. Adding 1.7 grams of psyllium to a serving of pasta had no effect on insulin or blood sugar in an English study.

Talk to your doctor before supplementing your diet with psyllium. It can interact with drugs that manage blood sugar, high blood pressure, or heart conditions. If your doctor gives you the green light to use psyllium, follow his instructions carefully.

Just one teaspoon, or about 5 grams, with water three times a day before meals can help reduce blood cholesterol levels and control blood sugar levels in people who have diabetes. Psyllium has no serious side effects. Just make sure to drink plenty of water. As with any fiber, don't add too much to your diet too quickly. Otherwise, you might experience bloating or diarrhea.

Shocking news about a popular supplement

Think twice before taking L-arginine, a dietary supplement advertised to put the "spring" back in your blood vessels and improve blood flow. In one study of 153 people who had suffered heart attacks, L-arginine not only failed to reduce blood vessel stiffness or ease heart disease symptoms, it may have contributed to the deaths of six volunteers taking the supplement.

Scientists say L-arginine might raise levels of homocysteine in your blood. Homocysteine can build up to dangerous levels, which can damage your arteries and lead to heart disease.

Previous studies showed that healthy hearts might benefit from taking L-arginine, but any supposed benefits for people who have not had heart attacks are questionable in light of the recent deaths.

If you have suffered a heart attack, don't take L-arginine — the supplement form of the amino acid arginine. You can get arginine naturally in foods, such as watermelon, spinach, shellfish, nuts, and turkey.

6 secrets to buying safe and effective supplements

"Natural" products are not always harmless and wholesome. Although many supplements have health benefits, not everything for sale is safe and effective. Your best defense is to uncover the risks and learn the facts backing a product.

Know what you're up against. The Food and Drug Administration (FDA) does not regulate the safety or quality of dietary supplements the way it does drugs. Consider these key ways supplements differ from prescription and over-the-counter medications.

▶ New supplements do not have to be approved for sale by the FDA or any government agency.

▶ Supplement makers do not have to prove their products are safe or effective before selling them. Nor do they have to report complaints they receive about side effects and serious health problems caused by a supplement.

▶ Supplement manufacturers do not have to regulate the quality of their products. And they can make claims about a supplement's healing powers without solid scientific evidence to back them.

Supplement manufacturers are expected to regulate themselves, but that could leave you with a few unpleasant surprises. On top of that, stores and Web sites can legally sell supplements known to cause serious health problems. You may never even realize a product is dangerous since warning labels are voluntary, not required. And while drugs come with product information explaining their risks, supplements often don't, even though they pose similar hazards.

Get wise before you buy. Too often, sellers exaggerate the benefits of their products. Find out for yourself what the experts say about an alternative treatment. Look for these reliable books at your local library.

▶ *Tyler's Honest Herbal* by Steven Foster and Varro Tyler

▶ *Botanical Medicines* by Dennis J. McKenna, Kenneth Jones, and Kerry Hughes

▶ *Alternative Medicine: The Definitive Guide, 2nd edition,* by Burton Goldberg, John W. Anderson, and Larry Trivieri

A few Web sites offer easy-to-read, unbiased information about herbs, nutrition, and alternative treatments. For instance, the Office of Dietary Supplements, a department of the National Institutes of Health (NIH), provides information about supplement safety and side effects. Visit their Web site at *dietary-supplements.info.nih.gov* and click on "Health Information." Check out these resources for additional advice.

▶ National Center for Complementary and Alternative Medicine at *www.nccam.nih.gov*

▶ MayoClinic.com at *www.mayoclinic.com*

Read about the latest test results. You never really know what you're getting in a supplement because no one regulates quality. Testing has shown that many supplements may not contain the ingredients they claim. Fortunately, the independent laboratory ConsumerLab.com has made a name for itself testing health and nutrition products for quality and safety. They publish their results on their Web site, *www.ConsumerLab.com.* Here you can find out which supplement brands had the right amount of active ingredients, and which posed health hazards. You can read partial results from their tests for free, but to see the full reports, you must subscribe to their service the way you would a magazine.

Watch out for contaminants. Supplements could also give you more than you bargained for, including contaminants like lead. A respected independent lab found dangerous amounts of lead in both a brand of coral calcium and a memory enhancer made with huperzine A.

The good news is the FDA issues warnings about supplements as soon as they learn of potential dangers. Stay up-to-date by visiting their Web site at *www.cfsan.fda.gov* and clicking on "Dietary Supplements," or call the FDA's toll-free information line 888-463-6332.

ConsumerLab.com often checks for contaminants when they test supplements. In addition, they also publish recalls, warnings, and other alerts on their Web site. You can read the latest alert for free, but you must subscribe to their service to see old ones.

Sidestep side effects. Herbs, extracts, and other supplements have side effects, too, just like medications. Your doctor helps monitor your reactions to prescription drugs, but with supplements, you're often on your own. You may not notice a problem until it's too late. For example, kava kava, a popular herb to relieve anxiety, stress, and insomnia, can also cause liver failure. Several countries have banned it, but it's still sold in the United States.

Fortunately, your doctor can help. If you're considering a supplement or alternative therapy, check with her first. She can warn you about the dangers, help you watch for side effects, spot possible interactions with drugs you already take, and avoid prescribing medicine that could interact with your supplements.

Find reputable sellers. Sometimes the FDA and Federal Trade Commission (FTC) take legal action against supplement sellers, especially those who lie about the healing powers or safety of their product. Find out who's guilty at these Web sites *www.ftc.gov* or *www.fda.gov/oc/enforcement.html.*

Combat cholesterol with plant extracts

CholestOff, a dietary supplement containing a combination of plant sterols and stanols, blocks cholesterol's absorption into the bloodstream, lowering LDL cholesterol but leaving HDL levels intact. Consider this supplement the 15-cent cholesterol cure — proven to work better than dangerous drugs. This supplement has fewer calories than other phytosterol-fortified products, like Benecol and other margarines. When taken as part of a healthy diet and active lifestyle, it could give your cholesterol an extra downward nudge.

Net the benefits of fish oil supplements

Fish oil fights heart disease, cancer, asthma, Crohn's disease, and more. In fact, getting enough omega-3 fatty acids from fish oil could help save your life. Find out how – and discover the little-known powers of these nutritious and heart-healthy fats.

Your body can't make omega-3 fatty acids, but you can get them from foods or supplements. Delicious cold-water fish are the most famous source of two key omega-3s – eicosapentaenoic acid (EPA) and docosahexaenoic acid (DHA).

Learn how they help. Because omega-3 fats help fight inflammation, they may help prevent or combat many serious health conditions, while also protecting your heart. Consider these examples.

▶ Crohn's disease. A recent study of Crohn's disease sufferers shows that the anti-inflammatory properties of fish oil can reduce the number of relapses. The people in the study who took specially coated, low-dose fish oil capsules for one year had fewer relapses than the people who took an inactive pill.

▶ Asthma. Corn, cotton, and safflower oils; dressings; mayonnaise; margarine; and processed foods are all full of omega-6 fatty acids. These can make inflammatory diseases and asthma worse. However, foods with omega-3 fatty acids have the opposite effect.

▶ Cancer. Inflammation may interfere with normal cell death and produce DNA-damaging free radicals, leading to cancer. Normal inflammatory processes may even help the cancer spread. But fish oil is a potential weapon against these processes. For example, men who eat fish at least twice a week enjoy a lower risk of prostate cancer than those who don't.

Fish oil supplements also show promise against arthritis, cataracts, Alzheimer's disease, and depression.

Scientists think omega-3s may work with your body to produce substances that stop potential heart attack triggers. These natural chemicals may help keep blood vessel walls flexible and prevent blood clots in your arteries.

Best of all, these omega-3s may help prevent "sudden death" – death during the first hour after a heart attack. The American Heart Association (AHA) reports that 340,000 sudden deaths occur due to heart disease every year. Arrhythmia, an irregular heart rhythm, may cause most of these deaths. But EPA and DHA get into the heart's cells and help stabilize heart rate, explains Penny Kris-Etherton, Ph.D., distinguished professor of nutrition at Pennsylvania State University. And that may be enough to prevent the arrhythmia that leads to sudden death.

In an American Heart Association review, Kris-Etherton and her colleagues examined the research on omega-3s. They concluded these fats can help reduce your risk of developing heart disease. Omega-3s can even help if you already have heart disease.

Several large studies have noted what happened when people with heart disease got enough omega-3s. Not only were there fewer deaths from heart disease, but also fewer deaths from other causes too, says Dr. Maggie Covington, a clinical assistant professor of family medicine at the University of Maryland with an integrative medicine practice in Bethesda, Md.

Supplement a good diet. If you have documented heart disease, the AHA recommends as much as 1 gram of combined EPA and DHA daily. You can get some from delicious fish, but the AHA suggests you ask your doctor about getting the rest from fish oil supplements. Your doctor can help you determine exactly how much you should take.

Although fish may contain contaminants like mercury and polychlorinated biphenyls (PCBs), fish oil supplements may be cleaner. Studies suggest that the supplements don't have environmental contaminants and that nearly all products contain the amount of EPA and DHA claimed on the label. But make sure you choose the right supplement. Look for the flask-shaped Consumer Lab's Seal of Approved Quality so you'll know you're getting a fish oil supplement that meets its label claims.

Seek expert advice. Talk with your doctor before you try fish oil supplements. They can interact with medications for blood pressure, high cholesterol, and diabetes. Because fish oil thins your blood, it can also interact with blood thinners like warfarin (Coumadin), clopidogrel (Plavix), and even over-the-counter nonsteroidal anti-inflammatory drugs, like aspirin.

Fish oil supplements can raise cholesterol and may even cause arrhythmia in some people. Research also suggests that people who have an implanted defibrillator for a condition called ventricular fibrillation don't benefit from fish oil supplements. Finally, be aware that you shouldn't take this supplement if you have low blood pressure or an upcoming surgery.

Dodge a common side effect. Fish supplements can have side effects like gas, burping, and fishy aftertaste. "Usually that can be alleviated by starting at lower doses and working your way up," says Covington. Also, there are now available triple-distilled fish oil supplements, such as OmegaBrite, that are said to eliminate virtually all fishy aftertaste.

Straight talk about a popular supplement

When it comes to soy supplements and your heart, there's good news and bad news. But even the cloud of bad news may have a silver lining.

The good news. A recent study shows this popular dietary supplement really does have anti-aging effects, including reducing dangerous fat around the middle. If you're a woman struggling with weight gain, this may be particularly good news for you and here's why.

Women are more likely to store fat in the stomach area after menopause because their metabolism changes during the "change of life." Unfortunately, fat around the middle can be more hazardous to your heart than fat in other places.

In a small study, one group of women drank a daily shake containing 20 grams of soy protein and 160 milligrams of isoflavones from soy. Another group drank a placebo shake containing milk protein and no isoflavones. The soy group, which substituted the shake for another food in their regular diet, gained less heart-threatening fat around the middle than women who drank the placebo shake.

The bad news. After careful review of recent research, the American Heart Association uncovered the new truth about soy. As a result, they no longer recommend soy supplements to lower cholesterol or heart disease risk. However, soy foods, like tofu or soymilk, can still help defend your heart, but only if they replace less heart-healthy foods, such as meat and dairy items. Making the switch to soy provides more heart-protecting nutrients and less saturated fat and cholesterol that promote heart disease.

Herbs that raise blood pressure

Herb	Scientific name	Use
cacao	*Theobroma cacao*	stimulant
coffee	*Coffea arabica*	stimulant
ephedra (Ma huang)	*Ephedra*	anti-asthmatic, nasal decongestant
kola	*Cola nitida*	stimulant
licorice	*Glycyrrhiza glabra*	treats coughs and colds
mistletoe, American	*Phoradendron leucarpum*	increases blood pressure
rosemary	*Rosmarinus officinalis*	stimulant
tea	*Camellia sinensis*	stimulant

If you'd like to try a soy shake or supplement, check with your doctor first. Taking soy isoflavone supplements is not the same as eating tofu occasionally. In at least one case, large doses of this supplement – used to relieve symptoms of menopause – caused a drastic rise in blood pressure. Soy isoflavones, from frequently eating tofu, have been linked to other health problems, such as increased rates of dementia, in an important study using excellent research methods. Soy interacts with many drugs, may contribute to brain aging, and may be unsafe for people with certain health conditions, like hormone-related cancers.

New hope for people with heart disease

Coenzyme Q10 might be the most intriguing supplement you've never heard of. Also called CoQ10, this vitamin-like substance helps produce energy in your cells, including the hard-working cells in your heart. Some researchers believe a deficiency of CoQ10 might contribute to heart disease. Although more research needs to be done, promising research supports the benefits of CoQ10 for people with heart disease. Some people think it might benefit your heart health in at least three ways.

▸ **High blood pressure.** High-quality evidence suggests that CoQ10 helps lower high blood pressure, but studies have yet to prove it beyond doubt.

▸ **Congestive heart failure.** Both research studies and experts in the United States disagree on whether it works, but CoQ10 is already used as part of the treatment for congestive heart failure in Europe and Japan.

▸ **Statin side effects.** This supplement does not actually affect your cholesterol, but it may come in handy to counteract the side effects of statins. According to researchers at Columbia University, people who experience muscle pain while taking statins have low levels of CoQ10 in their blood. More research is needed, but perhaps taking supplemental CoQ10 can help protect you from muscle pain and muscle damage.

CoQ10 has also shown promise in exercise-induced angina, heart protection during heart surgery and for people who have already had a heart attack. However, more research is needed to find out whether CoQ10 really helps.

Check with your doctor before taking CoQ10 supplements. CoQ10 may interact with warfarin, blood pressure drugs, beta blockers, and other medications used to treat heart conditions. It may also interact with drugs for diabetes.

If you decide to give supplements a try, take them with foods that contain fat. This will help increase absorption because CoQ10 is a fat-soluble substance. Recommended doses range from 50 mg to 200 mg daily.

Solve the multivitamin dilemma

Don't throw out your multivitamin bottle just yet — even though some research suggests large amounts of vitamin C, vitamin E, and beta carotene may not prevent heart disease, heart attacks, or strokes. In fact, some researchers say hefty doses from supplements may even raise heart-related risks.

Fortunately, most multivitamins provide far smaller quantities of these nutrients than the amounts used in studies. If your multivitamin contains just 45 international units (IU) of vitamin E, 60 milligrams (mg) of vitamin C, and 10 mg of beta carotene, you may be helping your heart. One study found that a daily multivitamin reduces heart attack risk by at least 20 percent.

Check with your doctor before starting a daily multivitamin for your heart. Some nutrients may interact with your medications or aggravate other health problems. If your doctor approves, your daily multivitamin could help your heart stay healthier for years to come.

Good ways — and bad ways — to boost your metabolism

Can boosting your metabolism help your heart? Maybe, but only if you do it the right way. There are many dietary supplements advertised to boost your metabolism, help you lose weight, and lower your risk of heart disease. But most of these products contain stimulants that may do more harm than good because they also cause your energy factories, the mitochondria present in your body's cells, to throw off free radicals. Free radicals are atomic scale electric charges that release tiny lightning bolts when they encounter almost anything in their paths.

However, there are four naturally occurring substances – reservatrol, quercetin, Coenzyme Q10 (CoQ10), and alpha lipoic acid – that function as free-radical neutralizing antioxidants that also help your metabolism become more efficient or boost your energy. There is a substantial body of evidence that they also help improve heart function without significant unwanted side effects.

Resveratrol and quercetin are present in some foods, especially in the peel of grapes and apples. CoQ10 and alpha lipoic acid are found in traces from a few edible sources and are readily available only as dietary supplements.

Eating unpeeled apples and drinking a little red wine or dark grape juice may provide sufficient quercetin and resveratrol for maintaining good health. However, larger amounts of these and CoQ10 may provide increased benefits. A recent study showed that taking very large amounts of resveratrol, up to five grams per day, was not associated with adverse side effects.

Resvinatrol Complete, a muscadine grape juice product, has extra resveratrol and other antioxidants, including quercetin, from grape skins. One ounce of this tasty drink provides 100 mg of resveratrol, more than would be available in a large bottle of grape juice or red wine. Check out the product at *www.resvinatrolcomplete.com*.

Doctors in Japan often prescribe 600 mg or more of CoQ10 for their heart patients. Smaller amounts are less effective.

4 reasons to bypass red yeast rice

Inexpensive supplements made from rice fermented in red yeast contain a natural version of lovastatin, the active ingredient in the prescription drug Mevacor. But these red yeast rice supplements may not be as good. Here's why.

▸ The amount of lovastatin in red yeast rice supplements varies widely. In fact, some supplements contain so little that they won't lower cholesterol at all. And some supplements contain a toxin called citrinin.

▸ Research suggests total lovastatin in a full daily dose of red yeast rice supplements may be less than the minimum dose of 10 milligrams in prescription Mevacor.

▸ Because red yeast rice contains natural lovastatin, it may produce the same side effects as Mevacor, including dangerous muscle damage that can lead to kidney failure.

▸ People with very high or moderately high cholesterol shouldn't take red yeast rice because the supplements won't lower cholesterol enough. You also shouldn't take it if you've already had a heart attack or stroke or if you're at high risk for one.

Make sure you talk with your doctor before trying red yeast rice supplements. These supplements can interact with many drugs, including blood thinners, high blood pressure medications, and drugs prescribed for heart problems.

Berberine clobbers cholesterol — but there's a downside

The traditional Chinese herb berberine may help lower cholesterol, scientists say. In a Chinese study, people taking berberine for three months lowered total cholesterol by 29 percent, triglycerides by 35 percent, and LDL cholesterol by 25 percent. Even better, berberine is cheap. For about 70 cents a day, berberine could be a low-cost option in the fight against high cholesterol.

However, this herb may cause arrhythmias (heart rhythm problems) in people who have had congestive heart failure, and it interacts with many drugs used to treat high blood pressure and heart disease. Berberine also may not be safe for people who have diabetes, low blood pressure, heart disease, and several other health conditions.

Boost heart health with pycnogenol

Pycnogenol, a natural plant extract from the bark of the French maritime pine tree, shows exciting promise against four threats to heart and blood vessel health.

Blood clots. Your next flight may leave you with more than just jet lag. Flying increases your risk of deep vein thrombosis (DVT) or painful blood clots in your legs. That may have something to do with the low cabin pressure during flights or just sitting still for so long. But people who have a history of heart disease or stroke are more likely to get these potentially dangerous clots, and some DVTs are fatal.

Fortunately, pycnogenol may cut your risk of DVTs during long flights. Italian researchers found that people who took pycnogenol had better circulation and less leg and ankle swelling after a flight than people who took a placebo. That's important because leg and ankle swelling can lead to DVTs during lengthy flights.

Pycnogenol may also be a good alternative to aspirin therapy, especially if you're a smoker. Pycnogenol may work like aspirin to reduce the "stickiness" of blood cells, one study found. Smoking and stress can trigger the release of adrenaline, a stress hormone, which causes platelets in your blood to become stickier. This can lead to the formation of blood clots that could cause a heart attack or stroke.

Researchers gave smokers aspirin or pycnogenol, and then tested their blood two hours after they had smoked a cigarette. Both aspirin and pycnogenol reduced smoke-induced platelet stickiness, but pycnogenol did not increase bleeding time, like aspirin. And here's another benefit — a smaller dose was required to achieve the same effects.

High blood pressure. Two small studies suggest a daily dose of pycnogenol can help lower mild high blood pressure. In one study, pycnogenol users were able to switch to a lower dose of their blood pressure medicine.

High cholesterol. An early study found that six weeks of pycnogenol lowered "bad" LDL cholesterol in two-thirds of the study participants. More research is needed, so stay tuned.

Chronic venous insufficiency. Pycnogenol also shows promise in chronic venous insufficiency (CVI), a condition where the valves of your veins don't work properly. Blood has trouble making its way back to your heart so it builds up in your lower legs. In people with diabetes, this can cause tough-to-heal leg and foot ulcers that may even lead to amputation. But pycnogenol may be able to help.

In two studies, researchers gave daily doses of pycnogenol or a placebo drug to people with CVI. In one study, the people who took pycnogenol were more likely to improve than those who took the placebo. In the second study, people who took a daily pycnogenol pill also improved, but people who got a daily treatment of pycnogenol powder on the ulcer in addition to the pill were more likely to heal.

Pycnogenol may not be safe for everyone so check with your doctor before you try it. It can interact with medications for high cholesterol, diabetes, and high blood pressure. Pycnogenol may also interact with blood thinners, like warfarin and aspirin. What's more, it may drive down blood sugar and blood pressure and affect your immune system. So play it safe and get your doctor's advice. If your doctor says you can try pycnogenol safely, take it after a meal to avoid stomach-troubling side effects.

Ancient Asian remedy battles cholesterol

Revered by many Korean and Japanese people and eagerly sought after by millions of others, ginseng is often called the "root of immortality." While ginseng may not guarantee you'll live forever, it might help you lower your cholesterol enough to live longer.

How it works. Ginseng may push cholesterol down in two ways. First, ginseng contains sitosterol, a substance that is absorbed by your intestines and lowers cholesterol. What's more, some herbal experts think ginsenosides, ginseng root's most active ingredients, help your liver snatch up cholesterol particles before they can wreak havoc in your bloodstream. This could mean protection for your heart and blood vessels and a lower risk of clogged arteries and heart disease.

Even though past studies and reports suggest ginseng helps control cholesterol, results from animal research have been mixed. But a small study found that eight male college students lowered total cholesterol and harmful LDL cholesterol after eight weeks of taking ginseng extract. Because this study was brief and had few participants, more research is needed to verify the study's results, to find out if ginseng is safe for everyone, and to see how long its cholesterol control lasts.

Ginseng's powers don't stop at threatening cholesterol. This amazing herb acts as an antioxidant and helps keep your blood from clumping into artery-clogging clots. It also revs up your immune system.

What's more, this all-healing herb could also lessen stress, relieve fatigue, improve memory, increase your strength, and regulate your blood sugar.

Who should avoid it. As fabulous as ginseng is, it may not be for everyone. Talk to your doctor before you try ginseng. It can cause drug interactions with many other medicines and supplements, including those for heart conditions, high blood pressure, high blood sugar, and high cholesterol. For example, you shouldn't take ginseng if you take warfarin (Coumadin), phenelzine (Nardil), or nifedipine. Also, don't take ginseng with large amounts of caffeine or other stimulants.

Don't take ginseng if you have liver problems or arrhythmia (heart rhythm problems). And be aware that ginseng has side effects. It can also drive blood pressure up or blood sugar down, so it could make high blood pressure or low blood sugar worse. Ginseng may also lead to nausea, diarrhea, insomnia, headaches, or low blood pressure.

Smart buying strategies. If your doctor agrees you should try ginseng, get ready to go shopping. You'll find more than one kind of ginseng at the store, so choose wisely. If the bottle promises you *Panax ginseng* or Asian ginseng, you're on the right track. American ginseng or *Panax quinquefolius L.* is generally considered milder than Asian ginseng. *Panax ginseng* is one of the "true" ginsengs, not an imitator often passed off for the real thing, and it's the most well researched.

Recently, a major consumer organization found that most brands of ginseng supplements are as potent as they claim and don't contain contaminants. To make sure you don't get one of the few supplements that failed the tests, look for ginseng supplements that feature the Consumer Lab's Seal of Approved Quality on the container.

Also, look for an extract labeled "standardized" that contains at least 3 percent total ginsenosides – or 30 milligrams (mg) per gram. Ask your doctor how much you should take. Herbal experts recommend taking 100 mg once or twice daily. If you stick with standardized *Panax ginseng* extract, the twice daily dose should provide at least 6 mg of ginsenosides.

Keep the beat

Super solutions for a balanced life

Laugh your way to a healthy mind and body

Stress comes in many forms, and none of them is good for your heart. Road rage, traffic jams, noisy workplaces or living conditions, and high-pressure deadlines all increase your risk of having a heart attack. That's because your body responds to stressful situations by releasing hormones, like adrenaline, that boost your heart rate, raise your blood pressure, and can cause spasms in your coronary arteries.

Fortunately, finding healthy ways to cope with stress can help safeguard your heart. One study found that stress management techniques lowered the risk of a heart attack or other heart event by 74 percent. Just taking a walk or chatting with family and friends can help. But perhaps the most fun way to ease stress and help your heart is to find something funny.

Discover the "best medicine." You may think improving your thinking is no laughing matter, but humor can sharpen your brain. It helps keep you alert, increases your creativity, and improves your memory. Laughter involves the entire cerebral cortex of the brain and gives it quite a workout. From the moment someone asks, "Have you heard the one about ... ?" your brain goes into action.

When you laugh, you breathe more deeply, bringing more oxygen to your brain. This makes you more alert, releases tension that blocks learning, and increases your memory.

Turn funny business into better health. Laughter really is good medicine for both your mind and your body. Laughter can help relieve stress and improve your circulation, immune system, and mood. It won't cost a cent either. Discover all the ways it can help.

▶ Humor encourages you to keep a positive and hopeful attitude. And if you have uncomfortable feelings related to aggression or other problems, humor can provide a guilt-free way to release them.

▶ People with a good sense of humor tend to have less fear of their own mortality. That may be why they are more likely to sign the organ donor consent on their driver's license.

▸ Humor helps you handle stress. Laughing at someone else's joke can ease tension. But if you can find something to laugh about in life's most serious moments, that's even better. Humor you create helps you see a stressful situation as less threatening.

▸ By sharing humorous, real-life stories, you can enhance your social relationships. This helps improve your health.

▸ Laughter helps your circulation by increasing your blood pressure and heart rate. This brings more oxygen and nutrients to your tissues and removes impurities, helping to fight infection.

▸ Chronic breathing problems, like emphysema, improve with laughter, due to better ventilation and mucus clearing.

▸ Quicker recovery from illness and strengthening your immune system are two more reasons for "tickling your funny bone."

▸ Laughing heartily for 20 minutes equals three minutes of hard rowing. That's pretty good heart-healthy aerobic exercise.

Watch and read things that make you laugh out loud. The next time you're in stressful circumstances, imagine how a comedian would describe it. Staying healthy has never been so much fun.

Get a case of the sillies

The average child laughs about 300 times a day, but most adults only 17 times. Add some silliness to your life and find your inner child.

26 proven, practical stress-busting tips

Cut your chances of a heart attack by 74 percent — without drugs, surgery, diet, or exercise. The secret? Learn how to handle mental stress, which can trigger a heart attack.

When you're under pressure, your heart takes a lot of abuse. The anxiety stress causes can lead to high blood pressure, atherosclerosis (hardening of your arteries), and abnormal heart rhythms. In one study, people with heart disease drastically lowered their risk for heart attack with four months of stress management training. You can, too.

So how do you spell relief from stress? Use these tips and find out which ones work best for you.

▸ During stress, you naturally take rapid, shallow breaths from your chest. Try this. Rest one hand on your stomach. Then inhale slowly and deeply through your nose while counting from one to four. You should feel your stomach rise or move outward. Exhale as you count backward from four to one and feel your stomach sink inward. Repeat this five or 10 times.

▸ No matter how much you have to do, get at least eight hours of shut-eye. If anxiety keeps you from drifting off, get up, experts say, and do something relaxing. If your brain keeps racing, make a list of what's bothering you and then let it go until tomorrow.

▸ Do 10 jumping jacks.

▸ Take a vacation. Interviews revealed vacationers felt better physically up to five weeks after a get-away.

▸ Gardening not only rewards you with a prettier yard, but it also lets you get rid of some of those worries along with the weeds.

▸ Forgive and forget. Holding a grudge is like holding yourself hostage. When a group of men and women took a six-session course on forgiving others, they had fewer episodes of stress-related health problems. The health benefits of forgiveness were still obvious four months later at a follow-up session.

▸ Look at the sky for a minute.

▸ Think massage. If you're keyed up, your muscles can feel tense and sore. A massage loosens those knots and helps you unwind and sleep better.

▸ Put your worries on paper, and you might feel more in control of the situation. Some people believe keeping a journal helps them sort things out and identify possible solutions.

▶ Squeeze a stress ball.

▶ Get a little sun. A sunny day can brighten your mood, but only if you get outside. Walk to the mailbox or a friend's house and the sunlight will boost your melatonin, a hormone that buffers the effects of stress and can help you sleep better.

▶ Confide in a counselor. Counseling is a great way to get some expert advice when anxiety and stress feel overwhelming. Chances are good that your health insurance will cover it. Ask your doctor for a referral or confide in a trusted pastor, priest, or rabbi. Either way, you'll feel better after talking with someone who cares.

▶ Watch fish in an aquarium.

▶ Give up coffee. Coffee doesn't just give you temporary energy. Research found that people churned out one-third more adrenaline and had more stress on days when they downed caffeine compared to caffeine-free days. Your best bet is to cut back on caffeine or eliminate it completely.

▶ Get enough protein. You need protein even more when you're under physical and emotional pressure. If your body doesn't get it from your diet, it will steal protein from your heart, lungs, and brain. So provide your body with a steady supply of nutritious foods. Lean meat, fish, low-fat milk, and egg whites will "beef" up your protein intake.

▶ Savor a glass of water with a lemon twist.

▶ Eat complex carbohydrates, like bagels, whole-grain muffins, cereals, and fruit, for fast energy that will stick with you through the thick and thin of stress. But stay away from the sugary carbs, like doughnuts, candy bars, and cookies.

▶ Read a magazine or newspaper article.

▶ Get plenty of zinc, iron, and selenium. In a recent study, test subjects under physical and psychological stress experienced a dramatic fall in their levels of these minerals. If you are stressed out, eat foods high in these minerals, such as beans, crab meat, yogurt, steak, clams, and oysters.

▸ Get more B vitamins. B-complex vitamins are quickly used up during times of stress, so make sure you get enough of them. Foods high in this group are peas, beans, lean meat, poultry, fish, whole-grain breads and cereals, bananas, and potatoes.

▸ Do a crossword puzzle.

▸ Stock up on vitamin C during hectic times, since your adrenal gland needs it to make stress hormones. Citrus fruits, strawberries, red and green peppers, broccoli, and cantaloupe are loaded with vitamin C.

▸ Munch magnesium. A Yugoslavian study found that people exposed to chronic stress had lower magnesium levels. To make sure you get enough of this important mineral during stressful times, eat beans, brown rice, grains, popcorn, nuts, spinach, peas, corn, potatoes, oatmeal, shrimp, clams, and skim milk. Supplements are also available, but be careful – too much magnesium can be dangerous.

▸ Sing.

▸ Ask your doctor about valerian. This herb has been trusted to relieve tension for centuries. It's also a super sleep aid. For valerian tea, add one teaspoon of the dried root to a cup of hot water. Or take three 475-milligram capsules up to three times a day. When selecting a valerian product, look for the Consumer Lab Approved Quality Product Seal to make sure you get all the valerian you paid for.

▸ Learn how laughter, music, and prayer can help.

Simple way to keep your heart healthy

Brushing and flossing can save your heart, as well as your teeth. That's because the bacterial infections and inflammation that come with gum disease also boost your risk for heart disease.

Fortify your health with optimism

Study after study shows optimism can keep you healthier longer. Why not see for yourself.

▶ A Dutch study found that optimistic men were half as likely to die from cardiovascular disease, including heart attack, stroke, and coronary heart disease, than their less optimistic counterparts.

▶ One study on people who had undergone angioplasty found that those who scored low on measures of self-esteem, optimism, and being in control of their lives were two-and-a-half times more likely to have a heart attack or require another angioplasty or bypass surgery.

▶ A similar study followed people who had undergone heart bypass surgery for six months after the surgery. Researchers found that the most optimistic people were 50 percent less likely to be hospitalized again for subsequent heart problems, like infection, angina, or a second operation to reopen clogged arteries.

▶ According to researchers at the University of Texas Medical Branch at Galveston, happy people are less likely to have strokes.

But that's not all. Just as optimism fortifies your health, a lack of it may raise your risk of stroke. Researchers in Finland studied the degree of hopelessness in 942 men who had atherosclerosis in their carotid arteries. These large arteries, located in the neck, provide blood to the brain. Four years after the original testing, researchers again measured the thickness of the men's carotid arteries, an indication of the risk of stroke. The men who expressed the strongest feelings of hopelessness at the beginning of the study showed the most thickening of their carotid arteries.

If cheerfulness comes easily to you, you're very fortunate. However, if you often feel sad or depressed, you might have a chemical imbalance. This kind of physical problem can be corrected. Visit your doctor for tests.

You can also see a trained counselor or psychologist for further insight into your mood. Sometimes just talking about your problems can lighten the load and your outlook. For your heart's sake, exercise your constitutional right and pursue happiness. Meanwhile, try these tips to help you "accentuate the positive."

▶ Survey your use of language, and change it when necessary. Change your negative words and thoughts into positive ones.

▶ Surround yourself with as many positive people as possible.

▶ Don't allow guilt about the past to rob you of today.

▶ Don't worry about something that has already happened. If there is a lesson to be learned, learn it and move on.

▶ When major situations are out of your control, find ways to take responsibility for the things you can control.

▶ Look for something good in a bad situation. It will reduce stress and help you cope.

▶ Ask three people you consider positive forces how they maintain their attitudes.

▶ Realize that how you feel about something is your choice.

Popular herb linked to liver problems

Herbs can cause side effects and interactions just like drugs. Unlike your prescriptions, most herbs don't carry warning labels, so you may not realize the danger. Take kava, for instance. Widely used to calm anxiety and stress, it seemed promising in studies. But the herb has since been linked to hepatitis, liver failure, muscle weakness, and scaly skin, not to mention dangerous interactions with prescription drugs, such as sleep aids, antidepressants, and alprazolam (Xanax) for anxiety. Experts now strongly warn against using kava, particularly if you have liver disease.

Surprising stroke triggers

"Invisible killers" can trigger a stroke. Researcher Silvia Koton from Tel Aviv University in Israel studied short-term triggers for stroke in older people. Surprisingly, she found that many had strokes within two hours of a sudden movement or strong, negative emotion. Even activities you're familiar with, like a doorbell or ringing telephone, can be startling enough to act as a trigger. Here's how you can protect yourself.

Don't make sudden movements. According to Dr. Larry Goldstein, Director of the Center for Cerebrovascular Disease at Duke University Medical Center, you should plan how you're going to change positions. Don't bound out of bed in the morning even if you're full of energy. He suggests you first dangle your legs over the edge of the bed for a few minutes. "Move slowly," he says, "rather than rapidly."

But don't be afraid to exercise — it reduces your stroke risk. Just get your doctor's approval for brisk walking, swimming, or other activities that help your circulation and don't require sudden, jerking movements.

Tone down stressful sounds. You can't escape every heart-quickening sound — like someone yelling for help — but you can change your doorbell. Replace an ear-splitting alert with a soothing chime. It will still get your attention, but you won't jump out of your skin when it rings. The same goes for your phone. Find one with a sound that doesn't rattle you.

Learn to keep your cool. Koton also found that 13 percent of her study patients experienced strong negative emotions just hours before their stroke. In other words, a short fuse could mean serious health consequences.

Count to 10 before reacting in anger. Or take a walk when you feel negative emotions welling up. If you feel angry much of the time, visit a psychologist or counselor for help dealing constructively with your feelings.

Although she hasn't completed her study, Koton is spreading the word. "High-risk populations should be aware of the potential influence of sudden, unusual exposures to familiar activities and emotions."

Roll with the punches. If you can remain calm in the midst of chaos, you're less likely to suffer a stroke. It's the vein-popping tension that puts extra stress on your heart and circulation.

Researchers gave over 200 men a test designed to frustrate them. Those who felt stressed out during the test were more likely to have a stroke within the next decade than men who handled the pressure well.

Use humor to deflect stress whenever you can. Sometimes laughing about a situation helps put it in perspective. Or write in a journal. Put your problems down on paper, and you may be able to calmly think of solutions.

Keep moving. You're more likely to get a blood clot if you remain in the same position for many hours – like on a long airplane flight. This little-known stroke trigger is even a risk factor for young, healthy people.

Be sure to walk up and down the aisle or to the bathroom every few hours to help keep your blood flowing. And drink lots of water, not alcohol or coffee. Otherwise, you could become dehydrated from the pressurized cabin – another risk factor for clots.

Even if you don't fly often, try not to stay in bed or in a chair for long stretches of time. Plan to exercise every day – even if it's just a walk to mail a letter.

The thought of a stroke can be scary, but don't let fear rule your life. Many people believe that even engaging in sex can trigger a stroke. The risk is actually quite low, say experts. In fact, regular sexual activity can help your heart and circulation.

Ambush high blood pressure with close ties

Just spending time with a spouse or close friend can help lower your blood pressure, research shows. It doesn't even matter what you're doing – just being around them makes a difference.

This probably works because you feel safe and comfortable around people who are close to you. Oddly enough, one study found that even participants who weren't satisfied with their partners had lower blood pressure when they spent time with them – although the time spent was more limited.

Another study suggests that married people with supportive relationships respond better to stress than couples with a low level of social support. Researchers studied 45 couples and measured their blood pressure and other responses to stress. Men with supportive relationships showed a lower increase in blood pressure, as well as less constriction of their blood vessels. Women with supportive relationships had less constriction of blood vessels, but the increase in blood pressure was about the same.

Researchers say these improvements in stress response translate into less stress on your heart. So even after many years of marriage, make time to be together. Go out for a leisurely meal, take a stroll, or use mealtime to discuss pleasant subjects. If you are widowed or divorced, spend regular time with a close friend who enjoys conversation. Your life will be more pleasant, and your blood pressure could benefit as well.

Relax your muscles and ease your mind

Stress tends to get trapped in tight muscles. That's why holding on to stress can cause crippling back and shoulder pain. To release your muscles, try simple progressive relaxation.

▶ Find a comfortable position and begin breathing slowly and deeply.

▶ Tense the muscles in your toes for a count of 10.

▶ Release them slowly and completely while you count to 10.

▶ Next, tense the muscles of your feet in the same way.

▶ Continue up the entire length of your body, tensing and relaxing every muscle group.

▶ By the time you reach the top of your head, you should feel completely relaxed.

---

10 simple ways to slash heart disease risk

Try these tips to help lower your blood pressure, reduce your chance of stroke, and lose weight.

▸ Count your blessings. Optimistic people are less likely to die from heart attack, stroke, and heart disease.

▸ Get a pet. Pet ownership cuts heart disease risk.

▸ Eat lightly. Hefty meals can raise your heart rate and blood pressure.

▸ Give up grudges. Anger, hostility, and anxiety are linked to rapid heart rate and high blood pressure.

▸ Laugh more. Laughter relaxes blood vessels and increases blood flow.

▸ Stop taking naps. Naps may double your risk of dying from a heart attack.

▸ Spend time with family. You'll reduce your blood pressure.

▸ Walk more. You'll make your arteries healthier and shrink your risk of blood clots.

▸ Get a flu shot. Respiratory infections and fever can sometimes trigger a heart attack.

▸ Enjoy your favorite music for lower blood pressure.

Easy path to a healthy heart

Make a simple change in your daily routine — eat before 8 a.m. — and join the ranks of the healthiest people in America.

If you think you have no time for breakfast, think again. British researchers found starting the day off with a healthy breakfast before 8 a.m. lowered total as well as "bad" LDL cholesterol and improved postprandial, or after-meal, insulin sensitivity in women. But skipping breakfast can lead to higher cholesterol and weight gain.

Start each day off right with a healthy breakfast, like whole-grain cereal, oatmeal, yogurt, or fruit, and help put an end to high cholesterol. If you choose cereal, double-check to be sure it's really whole-grain. Eating cereal for breakfast seems to lower blood cholesterol and cut down the amount of fat and cholesterol you eat throughout the day. Whole-grain cereals, in particular, slash LDL cholesterol and boost insulin control – benefits refined grains don't boast. Remember, eating breakfast is one easy thing you can do every day to lower your cholesterol. Even better, it won't require you to take drugs or see a doctor.

4 ways to stop stress before it starts

Try these coping skills to put a stop to stress. You may be amazed at the results.

▶ Plan ahead. If you're worried about an upcoming event, ask yourself what are the worst things that could happen. For each possibility, make a plan to prevent it and a second plan for how you'll manage if it happens anyway.

▶ Change perspective. When faced with a bad situation, find something good about it. You can also try this – instead of calling a difficulty a "problem," label it a "challenge."

▶ Figure your odds. If you're stressing about something that might occur, ask yourself, "Would a Las Vegas odds maker give this good odds of happening?"

▶ Take the long view. Ask yourself, "Will this matter 10 years from now?"

Music keeps blood pressure in tune

Putting a song in your heart could help protect it. That's because listening to enjoyable music not only relaxes your body, it can lower your blood pressure, too.

Often, before undergoing surgery, your blood pressure builds to a crescendo because you're nervous. A recent study found that music helped older people relax before and during surgery. In fact, when people in the study listened to music, their blood pressure levels went back to normal. It didn't even matter which type of music — symphony, big band, or even rock and roll. As long as they got to pick the music themselves, it seemed to work. The music made them feel more in control of the situation and helped distract them from what was happening. If music can help lower blood pressure in a surgical setting, why not during other stressful times?

Try music the next time you feel stressed. Also, try to spend time each day soaking up the sounds of your favorite tunes. It might put your life, and your blood pressure, back in harmony.

Uncover a hidden threat to your heart

Sleep apnea is a killer that strikes after midnight, but eight out of 10 people with sleep apnea don't even know they have it. That's downright dangerous, considering you actually stop breathing when you have an attack. Your windpipe gets blocked, and you wake up gasping for air — sometimes hundreds of times a night. This start-stop breathing puts you at greater risk for both stroke and heart disease.

It might not be easy to tell if you suffer from sleep apnea, but it's more likely if you're a heavy snorer. Experts have pieced together several clues to help you figure out if you have a problem.

Check for signature sounds. One of the best ways to uncover sleep apnea is to listen for its distinctive noises. At first, an attack sounds just like the typical rattling snore. But without warning, you start to gag and choke, as you struggle to breathe. After several moments, you catch your breath and return to snoring like nothing happened. Ask your loved ones if they've heard this pattern during the night. Or, if you sleep alone, tape yourself for a few nights, and see if you hear it.

Know these warning signs. In a recent study from Dartmouth University, two-thirds of people who frequently had morning headaches also had sleep apnea. And eight out of 10 headache sufferers who also snored turned up with the sleep disorder. Sleep apnea seems to cause these headaches by cutting off oxygen to your brain, so it's important to treat the problem and get your breathing back to normal.

Ask your doctor about cluster headaches. If your headaches come at night, that might be another clue, particularly if they're cluster headaches. These excruciating headaches that pierce one side of your head could be another symptom of sleep apnea's oxygen cut-off. Cluster attacks usually wake you up in the middle of the night, but they can strike in the morning, too.

Keep track of bathroom breaks. Stumbling to the bathroom late at night is not always a side effect of getting older. It could mean you have sleep apnea. A small study at the University of Alabama at Birmingham found a strong association between sleep apnea and nocturia, the urge to urinate at night.

Recognize your risk after menopause. Twice as many post-menopausal women have sleep apnea as do premenopausal women. If you are postmenopausal and spot one of the other sleep apnea signals, you have a doubly good reason to talk with your doctor. She could recommend treatments geared just for you, like hormone replacement therapy (HRT).

Fight back. If you suspect you have sleep apnea for any of these reasons, start your recovery by trying one of these simple lifestyle changes.

▸ Lose weight.

▸ Avoid alcohol and other sedatives before bedtime.

▸ Quit smoking.

▸ Sleep on your side instead of your back, with your face angled slightly downward. This helps prevent the most common cause of sleep apnea and snoring, the tissue of your soft palate hanging down and obstructing your airway when you relax after falling asleep.

At the same time, talk with your doctor about the best way to proceed. Since sleep apnea is a potentially dangerous condition, you may need to be tested in a sleep center for an accurate diagnosis. That could be your first step toward reducing your risk, sleeping more peacefully through the night, and waking refreshed every morning.

Approach Mondays with caution

Many people dread Monday mornings already. But now they have two more reasons.

▶ Mondays can be hazardous to your health, even after you've retired, a study suggests. A type of arrhythmia that can cause sudden death occurs more often on Monday mornings than any other time. Researchers speculate that the pressure of going to work on Monday increases your production of the stress hormones that may trigger arrhythmias. Over the years, this establishes a pattern that lasts beyond retirement.

▶ Research shows that more strokes occur on Monday than on any other day. This may happen because many people tend to drink and smoke more on the weekends. The stress of going back to work on Monday morning could also be a factor.

If you are at risk for a stroke or arrhythmia, avoid smoking and drinking heavily on the weekends, and learn to reduce your Monday morning stress.

Fight depression to cut stroke risk

Take steps to pull yourself out of the dumps, and you'll cut your risk of stroke. It's true. Experts say you're more likely to have a stroke if you're depressed.

Although the blues don't directly cause a stroke, the exact relationship is still a little fuzzy. Some people think depression causes high blood pressure, which in turn increases your risk of stroke. Others believe negative thinking, anxiety, and other symptoms of depression relate to a chemical imbalance associated with stroke.

Whatever the reason, there's no arguing with the statistics. A history of depression means you're 73 percent more likely to have a stroke. Depression may also raise your risk of heart attack.

Make some changes. To overcome major depression, you probably need professional help. This usually involves cognitive behavioral therapy, antidepressants, or a combination of both treatments. But for cases of mild to moderate depression, there are effective, self-help remedies. These can work if you are moderately depressed or just have the everyday "blues."

▸ talk with your spouse or other loved ones

▸ listen to music

▸ set short-term goals

▸ pray or meditate

▸ start a hobby

▸ exercise

▸ eat a healthy breakfast

▸ get eight hours of sleep

▸ join a support group

Watch what you eat. Also, consider changing your diet if you're experiencing sleep disorders, weight change, headaches, digestive problems, lowered sex drive, fatigue, worry, forgetfulness, or trouble concentrating. Depression triggered by nutritional deficiencies can bring on all these symptoms. But getting the right nutrients can lift your spirits and brighten your day, too.

Beat the blues with Bs. Believe it or not, a sweet potato or a spinach salad might help you. Both are rich in folate and pyridoxine (vitamin B6). Deficiencies in these B vitamins can bring on symptoms of depression, experts believe. Vitamin B6 keeps your brain's neurotransmitters in balance. These chemicals control whether you feel depressed, anxious, or on a steady keel. Eat chicken and other meats for B6. Plant sources include navy beans, sweet potatoes, spinach, and bananas.

Low folate levels in your body can deepen depression, but high folate can help defeat it. You'll find folate in spinach, asparagus, and avocados, and many other fruits and vegetables.

Depression can also signal a deficiency in thiamin (vitamin B1). Punch up your thiamin levels with whole-wheat breads, meats, black beans, and watermelon. These foods might help you feel more clear-headed and energetic.

Iron out the blahs. Beating the blues might be as easy as eating iron-rich foods if you have iron-deficiency anemia. Over 2 billion people have this condition and even more live with less serious iron deficiency. A sour mood is a major symptom of a lack of iron. Other symptoms include pale skin, sluggishness, and trouble concentrating.

Iron-deficiency anemia often attacks premenopausal women, people who regularly take nonsteroidal anti-inflammatory drugs (NSAIDs), and others at risk for chronic blood loss. Visit your doctor if you suspect you're anemic.

To get more iron, eat meat, legumes, fortified cereals, quinoa, kale, and other green leafy vegetables. To help your body absorb the iron, top these foods with a rich source of vitamin C, like lemon juice.

Find serenity with selenium. People who don't eat enough selenium-rich foods tend to be grumpier than people with a high intake, according to recent research. Eat some high selenium foods – like seafood, poultry, mushrooms, sea vegetables, and wheat – and feel the effects for yourself.

Cap off with carbs. If stress gets you down, a diet rich in carbohydrates might help. Eating mostly carbohydrates during the day, suggests a European study, may make stressful situations more bearable for some people.

The carbohydrate diet appears to work by raising the level of tryptophan in your brain. Tryptophan is the amino acid your body needs to make serotonin, the "happy" neurotransmitter.

But remember, choose your carbs wisely. Nutritionally speaking, carbohydrates from fruits, vegetables, and whole grains and cereals are best. They'll save you from stress and boost your levels of vitamins, minerals, and fiber.

Fight heart disease with restful ZZZs

If you're not sleeping well at night, examine your lifestyle choices. You could be affecting your shut-eye and your heart health. Try these easy tips for sound and restful sleep every night.

▸ Keep your bedroom cool and dark.

▸ Ask your doctor if any of your medications can cause you to stay awake.

▸ Stick to a regular sleep schedule, or regular time for going to bed and getting up, even on the weekends.

▸ Don't nap in the late afternoon or evening.

▸ Avoid alcohol in the evening. It can raise your blood pressure and keep you awake.

▸ Don't live in your bed. Use it only for sleeping and sex.

▸ Avoid too much caffeine, especially in the evenings. Caffeine can cause palpitations and rapid heartbeat.

▸ Eat a light snack near bedtime, but don't fill up with a heavy meal too late in the day.

Kick the habit with some help

You know you should quit smoking — but that's easier said than done. Cigarettes contain nicotine, a highly addictive drug. Nicotine has effects similar to cocaine, heroin, and marijuana, increasing the levels of the brain chemical dopamine, which affects the pleasure centers in the brain.

Willpower alone may not be enough to beat this addiction. Fortunately, you can try several nicotine replacement products that help make quitting more manageable. These include over-the-counter nicotine gums, lozenges, and patches — as well as prescription nasal sprays and inhalers.

These products help satisfy your nicotine craving without the added danger of tobacco. For example, nicotine patches deliver a constant dose of nicotine into your bloodstream. To gradually wean yourself off nicotine, you switch to lower-dose patches over the course of several weeks.

Gums and lozenges also help you overcome nicotine cravings. Just be careful you don't become dependent on them. You don't want to trade one addiction for another.

15 ways to stop smoking more easily

Smoking not only causes lung cancer, but it doubles your risk of heart disease. It may also cause up to 120,000 deaths from heart disease every year. Smokers are also twice as likely as nonsmokers to suffer a stroke. Fortunately, quitting dramatically slashes your risk of stroke and heart attack. In fact, within several years of quitting, a smoker's chances of having a heart attack are almost the same as someone who never smoked. If you're ready to quit smoking, try these tips.

▶ Read and listen to stories of other people who have success-fully quit.

▶ Tell your family and friends you are quitting and ask for their support.

▶ Quit when you feel you are ready and on your own time schedule. Try to pick a time when you won't be particularly stressed by special events, such as a wedding or an important business project.

▶ Get rid of your smoking stuff, like ashtrays and lighters.

▶ Notice when and where you smoke and plan ways to stop. If you normally smoke after a meal, plan an after-eating activity to distract you. Take a walk, do the dishes, or plan some other action that breaks the habit of your smoking routine.

▶ Write down all the reasons you want to quit on index cards and carry them with you. When you are tempted to smoke, read the cards.

▶ Plan ahead. Think up a bunch of stalling tactics so you won't automatically grab a cigar or cigarette when a craving strikes. If you can delay long enough, the craving might pass. Good stalling techniques include washing your hands, taking a short walk, or taking 10 slow deep breaths. Even fresh fruit can help you quit. Keep lots of fresh fruits and veggies around to munch on. Carrot sticks, apples, and celery are good choices.

▶ Make sure your first nonsmoking day is very busy, so you will be less tempted to think about smoking. If possible, plan to spend much of your day in places where smoking is not allowed.

▶ Pick a substitute if you miss having something in your mouth. The lollipop is a time-honored substitute, but you can also use toothpicks, cinnamon sticks, or sugar-free gum.

▶ Avoid wine and beer and you may be less likely to smoke.

▶ Avoid caffeine. Caffeine may increase your craving for nicotine.

▶ Indulge yourself in lots of warm baths or showers.

▶ Have the inside of your car and the inside of your house cleaned to remove the residue of smoke.

▶ Keep your hands busy with a new or old hobby.

▶ Think of yourself as a nonsmoker.

Remember – quitting smoking is a process. Don't give up if you don't manage to quit the first time.

Guard your health with a pet

You always suspected pets were good for your health, and now there's proof. Studies show playing with a pet can lower your blood pressure, relieve stress, and put you in a better mood.

For example, one study looked at 48 male and female stockbrokers who were taking medication for high blood pressure. When placed under stress, the blood pressure of those with a pet rose, but only by about half as much as those without a pet. And it's no wonder. Cats and dogs, especially, offer unconditional love that can buffer you and your blood pressure from the hazards of everyday life.

If you don't have a pet, try pet sitting for a few weeks. You might discover they make great companions. But before you get one, remember to take into account the cost of food and veterinarian bills, plus the amount of care and attention the pet will need. For instance, a dog demands more time and energy than a cat. And if you're renting, make sure your landlord allows pets.

If a dog or cat is right for you, visit your local animal shelter to adopt one. Don't give up hope if they are too expensive or your landlord won't allow them. Some landlords allow smaller, less-expensive pets, such as canaries. Like cats and dogs, these small wonders can also be delightful and heart-healthy companions.

Uncover hidden cause of high cholesterol

Did you know high cholesterol could be caused by an underactive thyroid gland? If you didn't, you're not alone. A survey found that more than half the people who had been diagnosed with high cholesterol didn't know if they'd ever been tested for thyroid disease.

You could have a sluggish thyroid and never know it. Most people with hypothyroidism experience weight gain, dry skin, brittle nails, and fatigue. But many older women have a low-performing thyroid without any symptoms.

If your thyroid is on the blitz, you may have high cholesterol and high blood pressure — plus higher odds of developing heart disease. See your doctor. A blood test can determine if your thyroid is functioning properly.

Put your worries to rest with prayer

When times get tough, the tough start praying. A recent study shows at least 96 percent of older adults use prayer to deal with stress.

What is it about prayer that makes it so effective? Dr. Harold Koenig, director of the Center for the Study of Religion/Spirituality and Health at Duke University, suggests prayer goes beyond physical relaxation. "The sense that God deeply cares about a person and is in control of everything that happens to them provides comfort that penetrates into all other areas of life and endures over time."

When unexpected events come your way, you may notice your heart races, your muscles tense, and your senses sharpen. This reaction is called the stress response. If this heightened alert lasts too long, your immune system weakens and stress chemicals build up in your body.

To counteract the stress response and bring on the relaxation response, experts recommend tai chi, biofeedback, or meditation. Now, many experts say prayer is just as effective.

Actually, prayer and meditation have a lot in common. They both can help you:

▶ Maintain a positive attitude. By praying or meditating, you can take the sting out of daily events that would otherwise send you into a tizzy.

▶ Live in the moment. In Matthew 6:34, the Bible tells us not to worry about tomorrow, since it will take care of itself. Living each day as it comes is a central theme in both prayer and meditation. Concentrate on the present through prayer to automatically knock out a major cause of stress.

▶ Focus on one subject. When you pray, you choose to set your eyes on God. You may wonder at his power, respect his holiness, or give thanks for his love. By focusing on one thing, the jumble of daily frustrations and events melts away, and your body can relax.

▶ Find wonder in the routine. While meditating, you may note the simple satisfaction of everyday activities, like cleaning the house or watering the yard. Koenig says devout believers often view the changing of the seasons with awe and delight – taking pleasure in the natural world as a gift from God. When you can glory in smelling the flowers, you pay homage to every moment of life.

▶ Use reason instead of reaction as you slow down. Prayer teaches you to see your life as God sees it. With his support, you know you will have the strength to face anything that comes your way.

▶ Make peace with the past. Forgiveness is an important key to any stress-release program. Doctors and religious leaders both agree – freeing yourself from bitterness about the past helps you develop compassion for others, as well as an inner calm.

Meditation offers you immediate and short-term relief. But according to Koenig, the effects of prayer are much more permanent and satisfying. "I think [prayer] is even more effective than the 'temporary' reduction in stress that meditation offers," Koenig says. "This is because prayer involves a relationship with God and a relationship with community – which involves more of a person's world-view and whole life."

Praying on your own can be calming, and sharing the experience with others is also helpful if you have heart problems. A University of Pittsburgh Medical Center study found attending weekly religious services helps people live longer. In fact, religious attendance is almost as helpful in adding years to your life as regular exercise and statins. Of course, you shouldn't scrap your exercise program or medication – but a weekly trip to church can't hurt. So set your fears aside and turn to God in prayer, the greatest source of peace available to you any time you choose.

6 ways to deal with anger

Anger can send your blood pressure soaring. What's more, if you're the type of person who is constantly wound up, even an angry memory will cause your blood pressure to climb higher and stay high longer. Yet, studies show if you learn to control anger and hostility, you can help control your blood pressure. Try these helpful tips:

▶ Count to 10 before you speak. Or take a few deep breaths to help you calm down and relax. You'll also be sending much-needed oxygen to your racing heart.

▶ Keep your perspective. Don't ruin your health over something you won't remember next week.

▶ Express it – then forget it. Express your anger in a constructive way. Wait until you are calm and can say what you need to without exploding. State clearly why you are angry, but try not to accuse others. Attempt to bring about positive changes in a situation. But even if nothing changes, express yourself – then let it go.

▶ Talk with a loved one or close friend about an issue that is angering you to help you get a clearer perspective. Ask someone who isn't as involved to help you come up with a good plan of attack to solve the problem.

▶ Avoid negative people. Instead, seek out people with a positive outlook on life.

▶ Avoid the issue. Perhaps the smartest way to deal with anger is to avoid the situations you know will cause it.

If you can't find a way to relax on your own, seek professional help. Taking a few training sessions in anger control or stress management could make all the difference in your risk of heart attack and stroke.

Soothe stress with good scents

The research is out, and the verdict is in — aromatherapy can relieve tension and daily stress. To lift your spirits, experiment with these essential oils — lavender, bergamot, cedarwood, frankincense, geranium, hyssop, sandalwood, orange, and ylang ylang. Just remember, never place undiluted essential oils directly on your skin. Instead, dilute them in a "carrier oil," like almond, apricot, jojoba, and grapeseed. Here are three ways to enjoy the benefits of aromatherapy.

▸ Get a steamy bath going and add five to 10 drops of essential oil and 1 ounce of carrier oil. Soak for at least 15 minutes.

▸ Dab a handkerchief with three to four drops of your favorite oil. Whenever and wherever stress strikes, sniff it at arm's length for instant relief.

▸ A 10-minute footbath with hot water and a few drops of essential oil, especially lavender, will make you feel pampered and peaceful.

Secrets to keeping your heart safe in winter

Even with a snow blower, winter storms can mean big heart trouble. Experts say you're just as likely to have a heart attack using a snow blower as you are using a shovel. Apparently, moving the heavy machine around is as dangerous for people with heart disease as shoveling. Here's how to avoid cold weather pitfalls — and look after your heart.

Shed the shovel. Shoveling is a tough job even for people in great shape. Combine that with stress and a heart condition, and you have a recipe for disaster. If you can afford it, pay someone to clear your driveway and sidewalks during the winter.

Make shoveling easier. If you absolutely must shovel, make the tool do most of the work. Choose a lightweight shovel that suits your height. If the snow isn't too deep, use the shovel like a plow to push it to the edge of the walk. Try to shovel early and often, since it's easier to keep clearing light snow. Take frequent breaks, and drink plenty of fluids. Above all, listen to your body. If something hurts or you feel winded, stop immediately.

Take it in small doses. Many people wait until the weekend to catch up on chores, like shoveling. Others stay active between Monday and Friday, but turn into a couch potato on the weekends. Either way, these spurts of exercise are hard on your heart. Try to space your physical activity throughout the week.

Learn to love layers. Women who live where the temperature changes throughout the year have more heart attacks in mid-winter than any other season. But in parts of the world where the climate is mild all year – like Taiwan – there is never a spike in the number of heart attacks.

You can't blame this all on snow removal. Scientists say the temperature itself can be bad for you. Because cold weather narrows your arteries, which reduces blood flow to your legs, blood clots cause more heart attacks in winter.

Since you can't hibernate, outsmart the cold by wearing layers. If you get too warm, you can always take off a scarf or jacket. And skip the outdoor activities on very cold days. If you get restless, go to a mall to walk. Finally, keep your house well insulated and wear a sweater indoors whenever you feel chilled.

Coast through a storm. You know to stock up on groceries before a winter storm, but do you know to take a break? Changes in air pressure that occur during a winter storm can put a strain on your heart. Researchers say a reading of 1,016 millibars on the barometer – an instrument for measuring air pressure – is best for your heart. For every 10 points the barometer rises or falls, the number of heart attacks increases by 10 percent.

The moral of the story is to take it easy during storms since the barometer may move several points. You can catch up on your chores later.

---

5 steps to fend off a fatal heart attack

You might not think lifestyle changes can really do any good, but guess again. Just five, drug-free changes can cut your risk of heart attack and death from heart disease by a whopping 87 percent, research suggests. These changes even help if you already take drugs for high blood pressure or high cholesterol. Here's what to do.

- quit smoking
- eat a healthy diet
- maintain a healthy weight
- exercise regularly
- drink only moderate amounts of alcohol, if you drink — that means one or two drinks a day for men, and no more than one a day for women

Even if you only manage to do two of these, researchers say you could still reduce your risk by more than 25 percent. So why not give it a try?

Impotence: early warning sign of clogged arteries

Impotence or erectile dysfunction may be frustrating, but if you pay attention, you could save your sex life — and your heart. Episodes of impotence could be an early warning of heart disease. Here's why.

An erection depends on blood flow to the penis, so anything that interferes with proper blood flow can cause impotence. People with diabetes, heart disease, or atherosclerosis (hardening of the arteries) are more likely to have the problem. Because the arteries that supply the penis are small, they may be among the first to be affected by blockages that could later affect heart arteries.

In fact, researchers looked at test results of men who were impotent and found that 40 percent of them had significant blockages in their heart arteries. This is associated with an increased risk of heart attack, even though none of the men had symptoms of heart disease.

The men in the study were lucky that their heart disease was discovered early. And many of them found that when they stopped smoking or lowered their cholesterol levels, their impotence went away. If you're normally sexually active and begin having problems, see your doctor.

Escape little-known heart danger

You might feel like you're having a heart attack when your plane takes a sudden dip. But in reality, just sitting on the plane might put you at risk if you have atherosclerosis or other heart-related problems.

Experts have discovered that flying causes a serious drop in the amount of oxygen in your blood, a condition called hypoxia. The root of the problem is the low air pressure in the plane's cabin, which can be the same as standing on an 8,000-foot mountain. At such low pressure, your lungs have trouble filtering oxygen into your bloodstream, and your major organs get as much as 20 percent less oxygen than usual. To try to make up the difference, your heart pumps faster and harder.

For a healthy person, this chain reaction can bring on a headache, tiredness, and other annoying but harmless symptoms. For someone with serious health problems – like blocked arteries, heart disease, or a lung condition – hypoxia could lead to fainting or worse, a heart attack. The cabin's low humidity, plus your anxiety, dehydration, and sitting still for too long, also add to your risk on a flight.

Before you start checking the train schedules, consider these tidbits of advice from the experts. They can help you keep your wings and your health.

Get permission for take-off. If you know you have a serious heart condition, talk with your doctor before taking any long flights. Ask about your hypoxia risk and whether you can fly safely.

Refuel before you go. A Japanese study found a great way to keep your oxygen levels high while you're in the sky. Simply make time for a snack and a caffeine-free beverage before you get on the plane. But don't go overboard before you get onboard. Stuffing yourself could have the opposite effect, putting more strain on your heart.

Master relaxation. Being nervous about flying only increases your health risks during a flight. Learn ways to relax.

Think before you drink. Some people down a few alcoholic drinks to relax and get over their fear of flying. That's one of the worst things you can do at 30,000 feet. Alcohol makes it doubly hard for your body to get a hold of some oxygen. Plus, it'll make you dehydrated, and dehydration is another major risk factor for airplane health emergencies.

Clear the air. Smoking makes breathing oxygen a hassle, too. Cigarettes wreak havoc with the tiny arteries that take oxygen from your lungs into your bloodstream. If you smoke before you get on a plane, you'll already have hypoxia before liftoff. Bottom line — quit or at least don't light up in the airport.

Take a mini-vacation without leaving home

Stress can leave you feeling trapped and frazzled. But you can "get away from it all," even if you can't go anywhere. Here's how.

▶ Sit or recline in a comfortable position. Take a few deep, slow breaths and then close your eyes.

▶ Imagine a relaxing scene, maybe a deserted beach or a snow-covered mountain. Imagine what you would see, feel, smell, hear, and taste in this place. Become aware of the landscape. If you imagine other people around you, take note of every little thing about them. Pay attention to what you're doing, too. Do this until you feel calm and refreshed.

After you practice a scene regularly, you will be able to recall it during any stressful activity for relief from tension.

Index

A

Abdominal fat 235-237, 249, 276
ACE inhibitors
  how they work 50
  potassium and 53
Advanced glycation end products (AGEs) 141
Aerobic exercise 216, 221-227, 295
Agency for Healthcare Research and Quality 35
Alcohol 284
  angina and 13
  arrhythmia and 46
  for high cholesterol 71, 133-135
  heart attack and 11
  heart disease and 131, 133, 284, 361
  high blood pressure and 8
  stroke and 18
  weight gain and 311
Allicin 129
Almonds 82
Alpha lipoic acid, for boosting metabolism 327
Alpha-linolenic acid (ALA) 78
Alpha-tocopherol. *See* Vitamin E
Alzheimer's disease
  exercise to prevent 239
  Mediterranean eating plan and 280

  statins for 58
American Heart Association (AHA), advice on alcohol 134-135
Anemia 350
Anger 357-358
Angina
  alcohol and 13
  defined 29
  emergency help for 15
Angiography 23
Angioplasty 28, 30, 339
Angiotensin II receptor blocker (ARB) 53
Anthocyanins 138, 141
Antioxidants 118-119, 181, 183-184, 313
  foods high in 97
  for high cholesterol 119
  in blueberries 138
  in cherries 142
  in dark chocolate 135-136
Appetite suppressants 261
Apples 110-111
  antioxidants in 111
  for heart disease 110-111
  for high cholesterol 110
  quercetin in 110
  stroke and 111
Apricots
  for heart disease 127
  to fight aging 127-128

Aromatherapy 358
Arrhythmia 45-47
    alcohol and 46
    berberine and 329
    defined 43
    Monday morning and 348
    omega-3 fatty acids for 43, 78
Artificial sweeteners 211
Asian diet 116-118
Aspirin
    common side effects 61
    heart attack and 11
    stroke and 61
Asthma 321
Atherosclerosis 4
Atkins Diet 253, 255, 297
Atorvastatin (Lipitor) 54
Automated external defibrillator
    (AED) 27
Avandia 68
Avocados 86-89
    digestion and 88-89
    for arthritis 88
    for high blood pressure 87
    for high cholesterol 87
    for kidney stones 88
    heart disease and 88
    stroke and 87-88

B

B vitamins 338, 350
    biotin 197
    folate 179-180
    niacin, prescription 53, 59
    vitamin B12 202-203
    vitamin B6 201-202

Beans 114-116. *See also* Legumes
    antioxidants in 115
    fiber in 114-115
    for high cholesterol 114-115
    protein in 115
Berberine 329
Beta blockers 52
Beta carotene 185-186, 326
Beverages, calories in 294
Bicycling 244-246
Bile acid sequestrants 58-59
Biotin, target amounts of 197
Bitter orange 263
Blood clots, pycnogenol to pre-
    vent 329
Blood pressure. *See also* High
    blood pressure
    exercise to lower 237
    target levels of 7
Blood sugar, diet and 158
Blood transfusions, heart surgery
    and 32
Blueberries 137-140
    antioxidants in 138-140
    growing 138
    health benefits of 139-140
Body mass index (BMI) 249,
    251
Borg Category Rating Scale,
    The 221-223
Bradycardia 45
Brain function, exercise and 239
Breakfast
    for weight loss 298-299
    to control cholesterol 344-345
Brown bag checkup 64

Bypass surgery 339
  depression and 34

C

C-reactive protein (CRP) 20, 250
C. difficile 35
Caffeine 314
Calcium 190-191, 291
  healthy sources of 293
  high blood pressure and 160
  nondairy sources of 292-293
  target amounts of 191
Calcium channel blockers 52
Calcium heart scan 26
Calories 258, 274, 289-290, 299-300
  exercise and 265
  in beverages 294, 310
  in fast food 306
  in fats 301
  laughing and 258
Cancer 321
Canola oil 74, 75
Carbohydrates 256, 337, 350-351
Cereal, high-fiber 106-107
Cherries, antioxidants in 141-142
Chestnuts 296
Chinese food 305
Chocolate 135-136
  beneficial types 71, 135
  cooking with 137
  flavonoids in 135
  for high cholesterol 136

polyphenols in 136
Cholesterol. *See also* High cholesterol.
  exercise and 229
  high-density lipoprotein (HDL) 4
  low-density lipoprotein (LDL) 4
  margarine to lower 89
  moderate drinking and 133
  natural ways to lower 6, 70
  sphingolipids and 170
  target levels of 5, 167
Cholesterol absorption blockers 60
CholestOff. *See* Stanols, Sterols
Cholestyramine (Questran) 59
Chromium 261, 299
  target amounts of 181
  to balance blood sugar 181
Chronic venous insufficiency (CVI) 330
Cinnamon, health benefits of 145
Coenzyme Q10 325-326
  for boosting metabolism 327
  for congestive heart failure 43, 325
  for high blood pressure 325
  for statin side effects 325
Coffee
  for heart disease 161-162
  high blood pressure and 162
  stress and 337
Colesevelam (WelChol) 59
Colestid 59
Colestipol (Colestid) 59

Complete Nutrition eating plan 172-173

Congestive heart failure 40-44
  defined 31
  exercise to improve 219, 240

ConsumerLab.com 319

Contrave 262

Cooking, healthy methods 301-302

CoQ10. *See* Coenzyme Q10

Coronary bypass surgery 28

Cortisol 275

Cranberries 119-120
  for high cholesterol 119-120

Crestor 54

Crohn's disease 321

Curcumin, for congestive heart failure 44

D

Dairy products 189-191, 283
  calcium in 190-191
  fat in 193-194
  for weight loss 290-293
  healthy choices 290, 300
  osteoporosis and 189
  ways to eat more 194

Dancing
  brain function and 239
  congestive heart failure and 240

DASH diet 154-157

Deep vein thrombosis (DVT) 38, 329

Dehydration 225

Dementia, soy and 117

Depression
  bypass surgery and 34
  nutrition and 349-351
  stroke and 348-351
  tips to relieve 349

Detox diet 277

Diabetes, exercise and 220, 229

Diastolic blood pressure 7

Diet pills 260-262, 263
  bitter orange 263
  diethylpropion (Tenuate) 262
  fen-phen 263
  orlistat (Xenical, Alli) 261
  phentermine (Adipex, Ionamin, Fastin) 261
  sibutramine (Meridia) 262

Dietary Approaches to Stop Hypertension (DASH) diet 154

Dieting strategies 277-279

Diets 253-255
  Atkins 253, 255, 297
  comparison of plans 297-298
  detox 277
  for diabetes 158
  for high cholesterol 168-170
  low-fat 166, 297
  Mediterranean 280-284
  Ornish 297
  South Beach 297
  Step 168-170
  Unified Dietary Guidelines for 288-289
  Weight Watchers 297
  Zone 253, 297

Digestive hormones 274

Distilled spirits, dangers of 134

Diuretics. *See* Water pills

Dried plums. *See* Prunes
Drugs. *See* Medications

E

Eating for good health 213-214
Eggs
  high cholesterol and 166-167
  substitutes for 167
Electrocardiogram (ECG or
  EKG) 22
Endurance exercise 216, 221-227
Energy-dense food 253, 304,
  309-310
Ephedra 263
Erectile dysfunction. *See*
  Impotence
Essential oils 358
Ethnic food 305-306
Exercise 295-296
  bicycling 244-246
  Borg Category Rating Scale,
    The 221-223
  brain function and 239
  calories burned during 265
  cautions 221, 228
  cholesterol levels and 229
  congestive heart failure and
    219
  dehydration and 225
  diabetes and 220, 229
  endurance or aerobic 216,
    221-227
  fatigue and 238
  fighting heart disease 216,
    229, 239
  stability ball 235-237
  strength training 217, 241
  stroke risk and 230
  tai chi 243
  target heart rate 227-229
  to save money 243
  walking plan 230-235
  weight loss and 240-242
Ezetimibe (Zetia) 60

F

Fat absorption inhibitors. 261
Fatigue, exercise to reduce 238
Fats 212, 300
  eating less 301-302
  healthy 256-257
  saturated 212
  to lower cholesterol 72-73
  trans 212
Fenofibrate (Lofibra, Tricor) 59
Ferritin test 25-26
Fiber 92-94, 178-179, 266-267
  benefits of 178-179
  blood sugar and 274
  diabetes and 107
  for heart disease 106-107
  for high blood pressure 93
  for weight loss 93-94, 266-267,
    273-274, 288
  good sources of 100, 106
  in beans 114
  insoluble 92, 178
  soluble 92, 178
  stroke and 93
  target amounts of 179
  water and 266
  ways to eat more 94

Fibrinogen test 24
Fidgeting, for weight loss 303
Figs 95-96
    diabetes and 96
    for high blood pressure 96
    for high cholesterol 95
    for weight loss 96
    stroke and 96
Fish 85-86, 198-204
    calcium in 292
    contaminants in 202, 311, 323
    for weight loss 311
    get more nutrients from 201
    healthy arteries and 79
    high cholesterol and 85
    mercury in 322-323
    peripheral artery disease
        (PAD) and 85
    polychlorinated biphenyls
        (PCBs) in 322
    polyunsaturated fatty acids
        (PUFAs) in 199
    selecting for freshness 86
    ways to eat more 198
    with garlic 128
Fish oil supplements 321-323
    arrhythmia and 322
    for asthma 321
    for cancer 321
    for Crohn's disease 321
    interactions with medications
        323
    triple-distilled 323
Flaxseed
    health benefits of 77-80
    oil 80
Flour, refined 177
Fluvastatin (Lescol) 54

Flying, heart attack and 361-362
Folate 179-180, 350
    high blood pressure and 160-
        161
    target amounts of 180
Food labels 293-294
Free radicals 183-184. *See also*
    Antioxidants
French food 306
Friendship, health benefits of
    342-343
Fruits and vegetables 182-184
    fresh, frozen, or canned 140
    get more nutrients from 184
    ways to eat more 186

G

Garlic 129-131
    ajoene in 130
    allicin in 129
    as an antibiotic 130
    for atherosclerosis 129
    for high blood pressure 130
    for high cholesterol 128, 129
    in combination with fish 128
    to prevent stroke 130
Gemfibrozil (Lopid) 59
Ginkgo biloba 39
Ginseng 331-332
Ginsenosides 331-332
Gourmet and gourmand 312
Grains 176-177
Grape juice 131-132
Grapefruit 280
Grapefruit juice, statins and 55

Greek diet. *See* Mediterranean diet
Green tea 313-314
Gum disease, dangers of 21

H

Headache 346-347
Health Grades 35
Heart, basic function 2
Heart attack 9
  air pressure and 359
  airplanes and 361-362
  defined 10
  lifestyle changes to prevent 11
  procedures to prevent 27-28
  signs of 9-11
  tips to avoid 360
  winter exercise and 358-360
Heart disease 18-27
  C-reactive protein (CRP) and 19-20
  gum disease and 21
  impotence and 360-361
  inflammation and 19
  LDL cholesterol and 19
  optimism and 339
  Ornish diet for 163-165
  sleep and 351
  smoking and 352
  stroke and 339
  tests for 21-27
  tips to reduce risk 344, 360
Herbs 340
High blood pressure 7
  anger and 357-358
  coffee and 162

DASH diet for 8, 154-157
  diet for 158-161, 165
  exercise to lower 237, 243
  friendship and 342-343
  music for 345-346
  pets and 354
  pycnogenol for 330
  vitamin D for 192
High blood sugar
  psyllium and 316-317
High cholesterol 54, 283
  alternative treatments for 58-60
  berberine for 329
  cholesterol absorption blockers for 60
  eating breakfast and 344-345
  eggs and 166-167
  fibrates for 59-60
  ginseng for 331-332
  Ornish diet for 163-164
  psyllium for 316-317
  pycnogenol for 330
  red yeast rice for 328
  Step diets for 168-170
  thyroid disease and 355
High-density lipoprotein (HDL) 4
Homocysteine 25, 317
Hormone replacement therapy (HRT), heart disease and 66
Hospital Compare 35
Hospital infections
  C. difficile 35
  methicillin-resistant *Staphylococcus aureus* (MRSA) 35
  protecting yourself 36
Hospitals for heart surgery 33-34

Hypertension. *See* High blood
    pressure
Hypothyroidism 288. *See*
    Thyroid disease
Hypoxia 361

I

Impotence 360-361
Indian food 306
Inflammation 321
Insoluble fiber 266
Insulin test, fasting 25
Interactions, drug 62-63
Intermittent claudication (IC) 37
    PAD and 37
    walking and 38
Iron 200, 337, 350
    target amounts of 200
Italian food 305

J

Juice, fruit 126

K

Kava 340
Ketones 277

L

L-arginine 317
Lactose intolerance 292

Leapfrog Group 35
Leg cramps 37-39
    smoking and 38
    walking and 38
Legumes 194-195. *See also* Beans
    cooking 196
    for high cholesterol 194-195
    ways to eat more 195
Lescol 54
Lignans 79
Lipitor 54
Lipoprotein(a) test 26
Lofibra 59
Lopid 59
Lovastatin (Mevacor) 54, 328
Low-carb diets 253-255
    counting carbs on 256
    dangers of 254, 255
Low-density lipoprotein (LDL) 4
    target levels of 5
Low-fat diets 166, 297, 299-300,
    301-302
Lycopene 143, 186, 282

M

Ma huang 263
Magnesium 197, 338
    high blood pressure and 160
    target amounts of 197
Margarine, for high cholesterol
    89-91
Marriage, health benefits of 343
Meat 204-205, 283
    cooking lean 116
    health risks of 208
    ways to eat less 209

Medical bills, reducing 243
Medicare 35, 296
Medications
    dangers of 62-64, 64-66
    free samples 65-66
    saving money on 66
Meditation 356-357
Mediterranean diet 75-77, 280-284
Memory problems, soy and 117
Memory, exercise and 239
Metabolic syndrome, diet soda and 211
Metabolism, boosting 261, 327
Methicillin-resistant
    Staphylococcus aureus (MRSA) 35
Mevacor 54, 57, 328
Mexican food 305
Milk, for weight loss 290-293
Monday morning heart danger 348
Monounsaturated fatty acids (MUFAs) 74, 206, 257
Morton Lite Salt 154
Multivitamin 326
Music 345-346

N

NER/S 53
Niacin 53, 59
Niacor 59
Niaspan 59
Nicotinic acid. *See* niacin
Nighttime eating 299
Nonexercise activity thermogenesis (NEAT) 303

Nutrition, basic rules of 213-214
Nuts and seeds 80-84, 204-205, 296
    benefits of 80-84, 205
    choosing wisely 209
    comparison of types 82
    monounsaturated fatty acids (MUFAs) in 206
    ways to eat more 206

O

Oatmeal 103-105, 275
    beta glucan in 104, 275
    colon cancer and 105
    diabetes and 105
    for high blood pressure 105
    for high cholesterol 104-105
Obesity. *See* Weight loss
Olive oil 75-77, 283
    health benefits of 76
    types of 77
Omega-3 fatty acids 74, 79, 199, 257, 283, 311, 321. *See also* Fish oil supplements
    for congestive heart failure 43
    sudden death and 322
Omega-6 fatty acids 74
OmegaBrite 323
Onions, quercetin and 129
Optimism 339-340
Orange juice 126
Oranges 123-126
    cancer and 125
    for better memory 125-126
    for heart disease 124-125
Organic food 109

Orlistat (Xenical, Alli) 261
Ornish diet 163-165, 297
Overweight. *See* Weight loss
Oxygen Radical Absorbance
    Capacity (ORAC) score. *See*
    Antioxidants

P

Palpitations 162
Peanuts 83-84
    resveratrol and 81
Periodontitis. *See* Gum disease
Peripheral artery disease (PAD)
    37-39. *See also* Peripheral artery
    occlusive disease (PAOD)
Pets 354
Phosphorous 192
    target amounts of 192
Phytochemicals 185-186
Phytonutrients. *See*
    Phytochemicals
Pill splitting 57
Pine bark extract. *See*
    Pycnogenol
Polyunsaturated fatty acids
    (PUFAs) 74. *See also* Omega-3
    fatty acids
Portion control 259, 264, 278,
    286, 303-304, 307-308, 310
Positive thinking. *See* Optimism
Potassium 187-188
    as salt substitute 153-154
    high blood pressure and 159
    target amounts of 187
Pravachol 54, 55, 57
Pravastatin (Pravachol) 54

Prayer 355-357
Pritikin Plan 267
Produce. *See* Fruits and vegeta-
    bles
Progressive relaxation 343
Protein 111-114
    lean choices 112
    stress and 337
    target amounts of 196
Prunes 98-99
    antioxidants in 98-99
    for high cholesterol 98
    purée of 257-258
Psyllium 316-317
Pycnogenol 329-331
    aspirin therapy and 330
    for chronic venous insufficiency
      (CVI) 330
    for high blood pressure 330
    for high cholesterol 330
    to prevent blood clots 329-330
Pyridoxine 350
Pyruvate, for weight loss 261

Q

Quercetin 131
    for boosting metabolism 327
    for healthy arteries 110
    for lowering cholesterol 72,
      129
Questran 59

R

Raynaud's disease, niacin for 59

Recipes, high-fiber
  Black skillet beef with greens
    and red potatoes 269
  New Orleans red beans 270
  Sunshine rice 271
  Winter crisp 272
  Zucchini lasagna 268
Red yeast rice 328
Relaxation techniques 238
Restaurants 303
  ethnic 305-306
  fast food 306
  weight control and 304-306
Resveratrol
  for boosting metabolism 327
  for congestive heart failure 44
  for lowering cholesterol 83
  peanuts and 83
Resvinatrol Complete 133, 327
Retinol. See Vitamin A
Rosiglitazone (Avandia) 68
Rosuvastatin (Crestor) 54
Roughage. See Fiber

S

Salt 147-154
  eating less 148-150
  flavoring alternatives 146, 148
  high blood pressure and 147-
    148
  Morton Lite 154
  substitutes for 153-154
Saturated fat 73, 212, 257
Scams, for weight loss 262-263
Scent therapy. See Aromatherapy
Seeds. See Nuts and seeds

Selenium 337, 350
  for healthy heart 181-182
Serotonin 275, 351
SilverSneakers Fitness Program
  296
Simvastatin (Zocor) 54
Sitosterol 331
Skipping meals 260
Sleep 351
Sleep apnea 346-348
Slo Niacin 59
Smoking, quitting 352-354
Snacks 209-210
  ways to limit 213
Snoring 346
Snow shoveling, dangers of 358-
  360
Sodium. See Salt
  content in foods 150-152
Soluble fiber 273, 316
South Beach Diet 297
Soy
  flour 118
  for heart disease 324
  for high cholesterol 117-118
  for weight loss 324-325
  memory problems and 117
Soy supplements 323-325
Soybeans. See Soy
Sphingolipids, for healthy choles-
  terol levels 170
Spices 314
Spinach 161
Stability ball 235-237
Stanols 89, 320
Statin Effects Survey 56
Statin myopathy 55-56

Statins 53-57
  alcohol and 55
  alternatives to 58-60
  for Alzheimer's disease 58
  generics 57
  grapefruit juice and 55
  interactions 55
  saving money on 56-57
  side effects of 55-56
  splitting pills 57
Stent 28
Step diets, for heart disease 168-170
Sterols 89, 320
Strength training 217, 241
Stress 334-338, 362
  aromatherapy and 358
  coffee and 337
  eating and 259
  laughter for 334-335
  nutrition and 337-338
  pets and 354
  prayer and 355-357
  progressive relaxation for 343
  tips to reduce 335-338, 345
  visual imagery for 362
  weight and 275-276
Stress test 22-23
Stroke 15
  blood clot risks 342
  clot-busting drugs for 17
  CT scan to diagnose 18
  defined 17
  depression and 348-351
  exercise to prevent 230
  gum disease and 21
  Monday morning and 348

  preventing 17-18
  signs of 16
  smoking and 352
  stress and 342
  triggers for 341-342
  types of 15
Sunflower seeds 91
Supplements 279, 318-320, 340
  contaminants in 319-320
  information about 318-319
  side effects of 320
Sweeteners, artificial 211
Sweets 209, 284
  natural choices 210-211
Systolic blood pressure 7

Tachycardia 45, 162
Tai chi 243
Target heart rate 227-229
Tea 121-123
  antioxidants in 121-122
  brewing 123
  for clean arteries 121
  for heart disease 122-123
  for high blood pressure 122
  for high cholesterol 122
  heart attack and 122
  stroke and 123
Thai food 306
Thiamin 350
Thyroid disease 288, 355
Tofu. See Soy
Tomatoes 142-144, 282
  for high cholesterol 142-144
  lycopene in 143-144

Trans fatty acids (trans fats) 73, 212, 257
Transient ischemic attack (TIA). *See* Stroke
Treadmill 295
Tricor 59
Triglycerides 6
Tryptophan 275, 351

U

Unified Dietary Guidelines 288-289

V

Valerian 338
Vitamin A 187
   target amounts of 187
Vitamin B12 202-203
   target amounts of 202
Vitamin B6 201-202
   target amounts of 201
Vitamin C 184-185, 326, 338
   for congestive heart failure 44
   target amounts of 185
Vitamin D
   for congestive heart failure 44
   heart health and 192
   supplements 192
   target amounts of 191, 193
Vitamin E 91, 206-207, 326
   for congestive heart failure 44
   for high cholesterol 91
   supplement warning 108
   target amounts of 207

Vitamin K 188-189
   warfarin (Coumadin) and 214
Vytorin 60

W

Walking
   heart attack prevention 229, 239
   plan 230-235
Walnuts 81
Warfarin (Coumadin), vitamin K and 189
Water 173-176, 302
   benefits of 173-174
   bottled or tap 176
   dehydration and exercise 225
   how much to drink 174
   minerals in 174
   ways to drink more 173
Water pills 260
Weight gain, causes of 288
Weight loss 248-250
   appetite suppressants for 261-262
   breakfast and 298
   eating slowly for 252-253
   exercise for 240-242, 295-296
   fat absorption inhibiting pills for 261
   fats and 256-257
   fiber and 273-274
   for better health 248
   grapefruit for 280
   green tea for 313-314
   heart disease and 249-250
   laughing and 258

Weight loss *(continued)*
  low-carb diets for 253-255
  metabolism boosters for 261
  need for 248-249
  orange juice for 286
  pitfalls 311-312
  protein for 252
  quick-fix plans 262-263
  satisfying food for 253
  scams 262
  skipping meals for 260
  sleep for 258-259
  soup for 252
  strategies for 263-265, 277-279,
    284-288, 298-300, 303-304
  stress and 275-276
  thermogenic therapy for 261
  tips for 250, 308, 309-311
  tomatoes for 282
  watching TV and 259, 299
  water for 286, 302
  water pills for 260
  whole grains for 251-252
Weight training 295
Weight Watchers 297
WelChol 59
Wheat germ, health benefits of
  107-109
Whole grains 101-103, 177-179
  benefits of 177-178
  diabetes and 102
  food labels and 103
  for heart disease 101-102
  for high cholesterol 101
  for weight loss 251-252
  stroke and 102
  ways to eat more 180

X

Xenical 261

Z

Zetia 60
Zinc 203-204, 337
  target amounts 203
Zocor 54, 55, 57
Zone Diet 253, 297